THERE WILL ALWAYS BE A SUNRISE

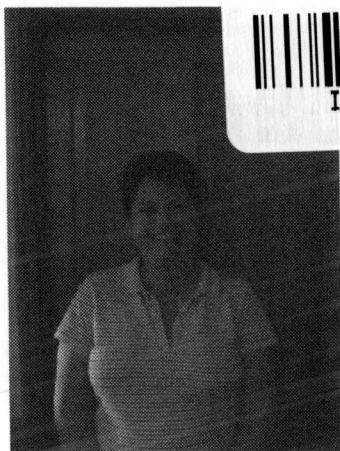

BY LORRAINE BLACKBURN

Published by:
Chipmukapublishing
PO Box 6872
Brentwood
Essex
CM13 1ZT
United Kingdom

www.chipmunkapublishing.com

CHAPTER ONE – STARTING THE PASSAGE AT IT'S END

Right that's it - I'm starting now, this minute, second even. Don't ask me why, I'm unsure of everything in my life at the moment. The only thing I do know, if I don't start writing now my brain along with the rest of my body will explode. There are only so many times you can go around the hospital grounds trying to march it off. If you have never suffered with mental illness, or even stress and anxiety, I guess you will be wondering what I am talking about. It's a long story but hopefully you will have found the answer to at least this, if nothing else, by the end of this book.

I'm 34 years old and have been told that I have experienced ten lives into my one. I know I have journeyed through thousands of experiences; many bad, some ok, others good and a few life changing, most of which I shall try to share with you. I have lived with poor mental health or bad mental illness whichever way you'd like to view it, since a teenager. I've had many diagnoses; nightmares/overactive mind as a child, bad premenstrual syndrome as an early teenager, anxiety and depression in my later teens and early twenties, closely followed by post-natal depression in the remainder of my twenties.

However the real big one, the misjudged/guided diagnosis that ruined my life for about 4 years and tormented those of my family is Congenital Compound Clinical Depression. These are not my words but those of my last NHS consultant psychiatrist who answered my question with this title when I finally had the nerve to ask what was wrong with me. So it is not a bad, albeit tasteless, tongue twister considering! My own interpretation of this title is that it had genetic origins, compiled of many complicated parts and was in fact a serious depression (I can vouch for that part). I remember very little of the actual happenings at that time, but the remaining feelings and emotions are available to me every moment of the day, if I choose to turn my mind towards that direction. My last and I logically believe, correct diagnosis is Bipolar Disorder, with an impulsive personality. Although I actually believe this is the way forward, even writing these words makes me want to curl up in a ball and sob. Why? I don't seem to be able to accept this diagnosis on an emotional level: it's as simple as that.

Writing this book, in a way, is extremely selfish. From later pages you will find I had (and still have) a passion for the sea and sailing. I am viewing this book as a sailing journey, or as us old sea dogs would say 'a passage'! I know this journey is going to take me through some calm tranquil seas, whilst at other moments raging storms and even unexpected, violent, windy squalls. I hope to survive all of this. I wish to bring some meaning to my life, to the pain, to the distress and at times agony. Amongst this I long for some peace of mind and acceptance of my illness, so that I can finally release the anger and move on with my life. Above all if I can help just one person accept their illness, let another know that someone else feels the same and it's possible to cope and educate someone else in the nature and emotional aspects of this illness. Ultimately being able to show that a peaceful dawn can rise after a wild storm, i.e. life is worth it. If I can fulfill any of these needs, then this whole passage will have been precious and priceless.

This is the second attempt at writing this book. The first was after I had been 'miraculously' cured, or so we all thought. However, it turns out that I was actually traveling through a hypomanic state. It makes perfect sense when comparing fact with theory but it is also equally disappointing. So all the wonderful, positive, loving thoughts are on hold for the moment, maybe there will be a sequel to this!

The other issue I want to meet head on is exactly that, this has to be completely honest - no bullshit. If not, it is of no consequence to myself or any one else. I don't want to hurt other people's feelings, but I have to write this as I see it, otherwise there would be no start, middle or end. We all view life, relationships etc in different ways, so that should be kept in mind. All I can honestly say is this is my way.

The style I will attempt is as though I'm talking with another individual. I'm hoping that way it will be easier for my thoughts and beliefs to flow freely, whilst simultaneously remaining personal. I am going to give some background information on Bipolar Disorder, as I understand it. Purely so the reader can keep this knowledge on board whilst following this passage. Hopefully, that way some of my actions, situations and experiences can be viewed from a wider perspective.

At this point I also need to introduce another dimension. Alcohol. I've had a deep and dependent relationship with it since my early teenage years and it has actually played a big part in my life. The more I learn about Bipolar Disorder the more I can see there is a strong relationship, which plays a significant role in a person's life. At the moment I adopt the label of a self-medicating, recovering alcoholic. Completely ironic - I haven't had a drink in almost 3 weeks and I have been in hospital for almost 3 weeks. Rather a strong coincidence! That aside I have been through detoxification and I finally feel physically dedicated to stopping. After all if I don't, the alcohol and therefore, the Bipolar illness will dictate and control my life. With the right support available to me (i.e. AA) I feel confident that I can solve this issue.

Yet again I guess this will be another passage through stormy waters, the outcome of which we shall both discover at the end of this book. Let's stay positive and keep looking for that sunrise over the horizon, it's the only option I have left to me.

CHAPTER TWO – RACING CURRENTS

I have actually managed to pick up three books on Bipolar Disorder in an attempt to find a succinct definition for you. Despite all my best efforts and resolutions, tears still sprung to my eyes, obviously, I'm not perfect by any means. I need to fill the sails with wind and get this journey moving. Right, I must return to the point but I expect this will keep happening! I don't want this to be a clinical reference book. Instead it needs to have a raw, emotional, human and comprehendible approach. So here goes.

Bipolar Disorder is also traditionally known as Manic Depression. I hate this term, repulse at writing it and despise saying it. The reason being, the words manic and maniac seem to cross over too easily. I strongly believe an individual's pain and suffering is real to them, in whichever form or degree they are experiencing it. I know I am not a maniac. I also view this illness as more complicated than just two mood states, in fact this label camouflages a multitude of overlapping symptoms.

So far, in a roundabout way, it has been established that this illness involves the individual suffering with extreme moods, both manic and depressed. We could get all philosophical about what is a mood, but that's not what this book is about (there are other texts that discuss this issue). I could just go on and on, but I won't, for me mood is a sliding scale of whether I'm happy or sad. It basically lets me know what my emotions are up to, creating a gauge (albeit steaming at times!), between the internal emotions and external behaviors.

Now for the next bit, mania and depression. My solution for this would be to get a set of spark plugs and during my next mood swing, I would connect you to my mind - no more explanations required! This way I would imagine you could experience the fluctuations of the energy in my mind, i.e. the highs and lows. However, I'm not Frankenstein, so the way I'll attempt this, is to provide examples of symptoms that I have personally experienced from each state. This isn't a medical appraisal but an individual viewpoint.

When I'm depressed I find it hard to sleep and I wake very early in the morning. I don't/can't eat, I feel a complete numbness about everyone and everything, I find it impossible to concentrate e.g. television, books and conversations, I become reclusive and no longer want to speak to people, answer the telephone and I avoid eye contact. I feel everything takes so much effort that I don't even have the energy to walk up the stairs, let alone make decisions. I have an extremely low self-esteem, am low in mood, very tearful and feel worthless and guilty about everything. The final and most dangerous marker for me, are my overwhelming, desperate suicidal and self-harm thoughts. These thoughts become completely intrusive and obsessive. In this state it appears that the sun will never rise again, but as I'm learning now, it always will no matter how cloudy, even if you don't want it to.

Now my hypomania is a completely different kettle of fish, but when out of control is equally as painful. Again, I can only sleep 3 to 4 hours but miraculously I don't miss it, I have so much energy I rush around doing a million different things. My kids think it's great when I'm 'crazy' as they call it. We rush from one activity to the next, full of jokes and playful comments. I also become extremely self confident /sociable and I have the perfect answer or joke for every conversation. I feel that everything is happening for a reason and that life will always turn out all right, no matter what. It's as if a higher force (I'm not religious) is looking out for and guiding me.

Then the problems would really start, my thoughts would race 20 paces ahead of me the whole time and that's scary. I would talk really quickly with words gushing out, often in a 'sing song' voice. Along with this I would become easily and extremely excited over the smallest of things. I would also start to become Mrs. Angry, becoming irritated when people slowed me up, got in my way or said the wrong thing. Simultaneously, I would become reckless e.g. spending loads of money without a thought and driving the car too fast. I would also start taking risks often of a sexual nature. I would suddenly have this insatiable sex drive, which has repeatedly led to promiscuity and affairs throughout my life.

I sit here now dragging myself up from a severe depressive episode, I know over the past few months, at times, I have thought please give me the highs back. When I reread these symptoms it shocks me back to reality. Mania is not great the latter part is hell. I was there last summer (it's now March) and diving deeper it was not a case of tranquil waters but more of racing rapids, which was bloody scary. I hope from these examples you have a better understanding of Bipolar Disorder, it was written from the heart and soul, not a textbook.

I have found a few interesting facts from textbooks. About 1 in a 100 people has this disorder to a certain degree. Also, it does appear to have a hereditary basis, although the exact gene (as far as I know at the present time) has yet to be found. There appear to be familial links to suicide, thyroid problems, post-natal depression and alcoholism. As we pass through this book it appears that I didn't have a lot going for me at the start! Now I think it is time to start on the passage of my life so far.

CHAPTER THREE – THE SUN, THE RAIN, BUT NO RAINBOW

Here we go. I'm actually scared of writing this part, mainly as I've already stated earlier, I don't want to cause anyone pain, but I have to write as I see it and with honesty. As a young child I have loads of great memories, wonderful Cornish holidays, fabulous Christmas times and great Sunday outings. I'm lucky as I am part of a huge extended family, which is all very close. I have two older sisters a younger brother and we grew up with lots of pets. My parents owned a general grocery store throughout my childhood and on the opposite side of the road my uncle owned a wine merchants with his family. My Granddad, a wonderful old Navy 'sea dog' lived at the bottom of our garden. No he wasn't a gnome, his property backed on to ours!

In my immediate family there are cases of alcoholism, hyperthyroidism and postnatal depression. Whilst within my close family suicide has happened, along with undiagnosed but suitably evidential occurrences of psychiatric illness. I haven't researched my family tree to identify other bipolar sufferers, as I feel that I know I have the illness and knowledge of previous family members will not change my life now, I just have to get on with it.

From what I understand I was quite a handful as a child, rather sulky, often in trouble and had big temper tantrums. The family had a poem for me, which I remember being frequently said. 'There was a little girl who had a little curl right in the middle of her forehead. When she was good she was very, very good, but when she was bad she was horrid'. It makes me wonder if this was the first signature tune of my illness, 'When she was good was manic, when she was bad she was depressed.'

I know that I was a bad sleeper, suffering from night walks and terrors. The GP put me on Valium for a while which my mum stopped as soon as she realized the nature of the prescription. I think this part of my life was reasonably peaceful in comparison to the future. My dad was a male chauvinist, he liked his meals on the table and expected mum to care for his every need. Mum on the other hand, rushed around looking after us lot whilst simultaneously working in the shop. She suffered with bad post-natal depression after the birth of my brother and always seemed to be living off her nerves. We were frequently told by her, "if you carry on like this I will end up in St James". Ironic really as that is the exact psychiatric hospital I was unfortunate enough to spend thirteen months of my 'life' (if you could call it that!). I would never use a phrase like that with my own children, it would be a million times scarier for them, after all it was a reality.

I know I would fall out and argue with my dad, we were never able to see eye to eye and had very few good times together. Looking back I think I first started having real problems when I was about 14 years old. I was a bit of a loner at school, I was ok at making friends when I was happy, but we always drifted apart when I was sad. This happy/sad scenario was extremely apparent, often blamed on 'teenage years', but as much as anything on premenstrual syndrome. I dare say both were relevant. I dedicated myself to dinghy sailing, had an older boyfriend (although he frequently put me down) and I just drifted along.

I know I used to spend many hours wondering over the meaning of life, what happens in/after death and when would the world end? I guess I was rather morbid. The first time (of many) I was drunk at school was around 15. It was St Valentine's Day, my boyfriend was away in the RAF and I can remember sitting in assembly with my head spinning. I'd seen my dad get drunk every single night from when I could first remember, so I just thought right, I'm so miserable I'll give it a go. I liked feeling detached, calm, numb and peaceful, I could go on. So I guess this is when my destructive relationship with alcohol began, which carried on throughout my college education and the rest of my life.

I went on to college to study A levels with the ambition of becoming a nurse. I never imagined that I was clever enough to take a degree. I studied psychology at A level, which is when my passion for the subject began to grow. If I was a loner before, I was an isolated iceberg here. My boyfriend was stationed away and the only things that kept me going were my sailing, the love of the sea and alcohol.

Before I enter my own turmoil I need to paint a picture of what was happening around me. My grandfather died from lung cancer and my elder sister who had married at 20 had left her husband. My parents' business had tax problems and they were entering the anxiety of selling whilst my dad was looking for a new career. My other sister, who always held the family together, was away at university. There was quite a lot of shit going on. I try to consol myself that these were the reasons for my dad's behaviour.

I also used to work in the shop, do the housework, cook a lot of the meals and do the ironing. We were all meant to be pulling together during this difficult time, a very good idea, but it left me with zero time. This meant little opportunity to study, no social life (I had few friends anyway), very limited time with my boyfriend and most importantly, virtually no time for myself. This is one reason why I think I went so wild in Bath.

I always wondered why my dad seemed to hate me. He'll deny the fact, but in spite of a few private theories, nothing else explained his behaviour and boy did I hate him at the time. What I've come up with is that he wouldn't accept I could actually, possibly be intelligent, after all it was only my sister Sue who had inherited his brains. My boobs were too big, my hair too blonde, I had too many boyfriends, I argued too much and I stood up to him too much... He often described me as a blonde bimbo, stupid or thick, as well as nicer (sarcasm) terms such as slut, loose, and tart, not to mention the less offensive ones.

Out of his four children it was only me that he abused in this way. I've spent hours trying to work out why and for the comfort of others, I will not mention some of the theories developed through therapy here. Finally, a few years later (my early 20's) my mum freely admitted that "Yes he does treat you differently, but I don't know why". This declaration was made through rivers of tears after yet another violently abusive outburst from my dad towards me. For me that was a huge revelation, my mum closest of all to the situation, provided validation and it was no longer just an isolated figment of my imagination. Life is different now that he doesn't seem to have the energy or will power to do it to the same degree.

As already mentioned Dad drank, normally Guinness shortly followed by numerous whiskies. All of us would avoid having anyone home if there was a possibility that Dad would be drunk, especially if Mum wasn't home, as he would drink more. His eyes would become unfocused, speech slurred, movements clumsy and if eating he just resembled a pig. For no apparent reason he would start shouting and flare into a rage. However, the most embarrassing of all, even in front of guests, would be when he did a running commentary of the women on television e.g. the size of their breasts and if they were worth giving a seeing to (I hasten to add that I'm using polite language for the benefit of the reader). The worst nights for me would be on Thursdays as everyone else would be out. Normally I would sit at my aunt and uncle's house, their house was a second home to me. One particular night was different which stands out amongst the many for me. I will explain the situation.

I'd had Parents' Evening, which my Dad hadn't wanted to go to (I guess I wasn't clever enough for him to bother about), so Mum (who had gone) went on to her Badminton Club without doing his tea. I had a huge piece of coursework due in the next day as my final exams were drawing near. I hadn't gone over to my aunt's house because of this. After a decent amount of booze my Dad had decided that he was hungry and told me to cook his tea. I was in a dilemma I HAD to get the coursework finished, but my dad was drunk. With quick thinking, I decided on a compromise and offered to show him how to cook his meal (after all he was such an intelligent man - sarcastic thoughts) and it was something simple. Immediately the explosion took place, torrents of crude, verbal abuse, whilst simultaneously physically threatening. Shit, this time I was terrified, not just scared. The next thing I knew he had a long sharp knife out of the drawer, which he was waving in front of my face as he swayed. I wanted to believe that he had no intention of actually using the knife, it was more to reinforce the verbal abuse. I just did not know. What makes a person step over that line and into the realms of taking a life? I ran upstairs through the top of the house to the other side, where I went downstairs and phoned my boyfriend. The fear was so great that I was frozen to the spot, sitting on the stairs, barely able to keep hold of the telephone because I was shaking so much. Then I heard his laboured breathing upstairs on the landing and the lights went out. I sat in the darkness for what could have been only seconds. It felt like hours before I was able to come to my senses and switch the light back on. Each time I switched it on, he would turn it off, it resembled a scene from a horror movie. What the hell was going on in this man's head to treat his own daughter like this? Suddenly I snapped and knew that I had to get out of there. I ran through the back door and just kept on going. I must have raced through a large chunk of Portsmouth. I was looking for my sister Sue and her boyfriend Andy. Eventually, physically and emotionally blown, I crept back into the house to discover Dad asleep in his chair and this time, although only hours had passed it felt like days.

I went upstairs through to my brother's room (we had adjoining rooms) and told him what the situation was. He came up with a plan. Paul put lots of cushions on the floor, therefore if Dad came through his room Paul would hear him trip. He also kept some sort of solid weapon (I fail to remember the type) in his bed just in case Dad came after me. I then headed off to bed fully clothed with trainers on, shaking and terrified but prepared to run if necessary. I guess this is a good example of the biological fight or flight response. Needless to say I didn't get my coursework finished. The next morning I was informed by Mum that if anything similar to the previous night ever happened again I was to leave. I was seventeen years old. Why, oh why, did she always support him? Was she just being submissive or was she scared? I have no answers. My elder sister was a non-entity, but Sue as always was there for me and said that if there was a repeat situation I could move into Andy's flat (he was a fantastic big brother to me).

I know this isn't all a dream (or should I say nightmare), or made up, and I know for some it is going to be very uncomfortable. However, it is complete honesty and the truth through my eyes. As already mentioned I am blessed with a large extended family. I am particularly close to another aunt and uncle and we have discussed these issues many times. My aunt has told me that from a very young age, it was so obvious that I was treated differently, so they would have me to stay a lot. They have always been a huge source of comfort and advice and I greatly value them and always will.

Life for my parents has changed a great deal over the past fifteen years. They had to close the shop and find alternative employment. My dad seemed to lose some of his dignity, pride, chauvinism, pig headedness and bullying tactics. Mum has also changed she has become more assertive, knows her own mind, stands up for her rights and doesn't worry so much.

I love my mum unconditionally, I always have done and I always will. As for my dad, yes I do love him, I have to, at times he can be good company and I'm no longer scared of him but I will never be able to forgive and forget. I just wish the past could have been different. I feel as though I've missed out on one of life's greatest relationships, that of a father and daughter. When I watch other people I can't even begin to imagine what that bond must be like, it is a complete mystery to me. The one thing I do know and can faithfully promise, is that I will never, ever, let him bully or speak to my own children like that. They are my precious sunrise.

CHAPTER FOUR – THE RAGING STORM

On achieving good A-level results I headed off to Bath to train for my Registered General Nurse qualification at the Royal United Hospital. I was so excited about leaving the bad stuff behind and entering a new free world bursting with positive expectations. Little did I know that I was diving headfirst into one of the worst hurricanes of my life so far. I can't write this in chronological order, to be honest I think it will take too long while you will find it tedious. At the present time I think I need to address different issues and the situations I found myself in. So cast the lines, we're off!

Friendships first I think. I was so excited meeting all these new potential friends and to start off with it was so easy to get on well with everyone. At this time I think I must have been going through my first proper high, but of course there was absolutely no reason for anyone to suspect this. As time went on and we all started on different wards, the hours became unsociable and allocations spread through different hospitals. People drifted, making firm friends with some and casual relationships with others.

For me the same old cycle began, which I have only recognized since learning about this illness. I made firm intense friendships, constantly partied and became amazingly social with brilliant communication and listening skills. I had so much energy, always busy and always helping others. Then BANG the depression would come, although I didn't know what it was then and the complete opposite would happen to my friendships and myself. Suddenly, I would find myself completely on my own, isolated, a recluse and regarded as weird. This cycle would continually rotate through different groups of people, most of whom were completely diverse from each other. I ended up moving flats so many times that I've lost count, but it was always with my new 'best mates', always with the view that this time would be better and always simply, because 'it seemed like the right thing to do'. How could my perceptions be so misguided? Was it due to the numerous highs, or the confused feelings on a low, with the wish that anything had to be better than this?

So, where did the depression spring from? It was more of a creep actually. The black moods that arrived around my periods stopped having an ending. They just wrapped themselves around each other (somewhat like the sheets (ropes) in yachting do when left to flap in the wind). I blamed it on the ward I was on, where I lived, the coursework, the people I lived with, grasping for concrete explanations. It was so scary I could find no secure, logical explanation and suffered dreadfully knowing that I had absolutely no control over it. This is something I torture myself with even today, the lack of control. I even left nursing for a 3 week period, desperately trying to make anything work. I felt so frightened, it was worse than anything I'd ever known, I could fathom no logic or establish control over it.

My tutors knew that I was having problems as they always came out in my written work, but they seemed to flounder and were unable to give me any direction. Eventually, I saw my GP and was prescribed antidepressants, the first of many. I can't really work out the order of all the accompanying effects the illness had, so it is going to be served on a huge plate for you to pick through. Leading on from antidepressants I became addicted to a rather large dosage of Lorazepam (from the same drug family as Valium). I managed to overcome this addiction, further down the road after my first overdose, with the support of some amazing staff during my placement in the casualty department.

I saw various professionals, most of whom were of little help. I remember one day in desperation telling my female counsellor that I was going to commit suicide. To which I received a "Yes dear we'll talk about it in two weeks at your next appointment". Now to me that was screaming for help but it still fell on deaf ears. I went outside and sat on the grass frozen for two hours, knowing that if I moved I would kill myself. In retrospect I dare say that she could have seen me from her room. I did in fact; try to take my life a few weeks later.

Maybe I should talk about how the depression felt, however the way it felt then is exactly the same as now; varying slightly in the way in which different waves lap against the hull of a yacht. During this time I also began an intimate relationship with an eating disorder and established the obsession of self-harming. I was obviously working really hard, just on the wrong subjects!

For me self-harming was not a cry for help, trying to bring attention to my pain, a form of blaming others or an attempt at changing another's behaviours and beliefs. It was actually the fact that I was in so much psychological pain that I had to do something to release it.

It was as though my whole being, mind, body and soul were screaming out in agony. However, there were no available psychological 'pain killers' for me to reach out for to comfort this torture. I now know of a psychological approach (Cognitive Behavioural Therapy) that has proven to be a fantastic eraser of such agony and I currently endeavour to use this in my day-to-day life.

I would hurt myself, the methods by which would vary greatly, iron burns, cigarette burns, black eyes, slamming hands in drawers/doors, cuts with razors and on and on. Each time I hurt myself I felt immense relief, pointlessly though as this relief was very short lived, minutes at the most. So I would repeat the action but with greater force and intent. My behaviours were extremely obsessive and impulsive as, I never thought further than those first few moments. Consequently, I would forget there would be visible marks and that I would have to tell elaborate lies to numerous people to conceal. This in itself just led to more deceit, something my whole life was now made of. I would tell myself 'tough you deserved it, now lets see you get out of this one'.

On my psychiatric placement I was taken to one side and embarrassingly asked if my boyfriend was hitting me, I had to make up some excuse about a door I didn't see. I had 3 more difficult situations during that placement. Firstly, I had to sit with an anorexic girl to watch her whilst she ate. Her words were along the lines of "I don't know why you're watching me, you're worse than I am". I was. Secondly, we (the student nurses) had to participate in the art therapy session with the patients, however I was the only one asked to remain behind by the therapist, due to my work being so disturbing. Finally, my coursework was based on a wonderful woman who was suffering with severe clinical depression. This led to my presence being requested at the school due to my work displaying 'rather a bit too much insight'. This meeting still failed to get me any help, maybe I was too much of an actress covering up my tracks.

Throughout all of these events I was also drinking heavily, certainly to a degree socially, but mainly as a lame attempt to relieve the symptoms of pain and fear. So what next? My eating disorder and the two overdoses, or do I say lightly, sexual abuse. I think the eating disorder. I first became aware of my weight when I was at college during my pre-nursing course. We did a sponsored diet on the excuse of helping a local nursery, with the purpose of 'tactfully' helping out a largely overweight girl on the course. I could really question the ethics of this now, but I guess things may have been different then. What, when, where or how I cannot remember now, maybe that's just convenient for my mind. All I know is that I entered a nightmarish cycle of control. I think that maybe the anxiety and distress caused me to miss meals (I still have this problem now), which in turn made me lose weight. At what point did it swap from a nervous tummy to making myself sick? If we were to draw a cyclic diagram now, I think I would add an arrow saying control.

The depression and mania left me with very little control over my life. The illness affected all of my relationships, both sexual and platonic, my awareness of danger, my sociability and my professional and student life, so why not my body image as well. I quickly discovered that by making the decision to stick my fingers down my throat to induce vomiting, I could return to a sense of control. I was back in charge or so I thought. Next I decided that I looked fat, which I wasn't in any shape or form, just healthy. So not only did I feel in control, I was also getting a buzz from manipulating my weight and this was like a drug to me. These feelings seem to be similar to those in a hypomanic episode i.e. I felt good, really good again, rather than depressed and scared. The next progression was starvation. My obsessed mind determined that if I lost weight from vomiting then surely I'd lose weight if I starved myself. I had a logical problem that if I didn't eat, what could I be sick on? It's amazing what small amounts need to be consumed (and this includes drinking) to still enable you to vomit for a good few minutes. However, this would mean I was unable to keep as quiet. To be basic, you end up retching. I can remember an occasion when one of my flat mates was banging on the toilet door, shouting at me to stop, but I ignored her and carried on.

I then progressed on to laxatives, I don't even know how I was aware of this next stage, it just automatically happened. The first time I asked for some at the chemists I made up a story that they were for my grandmother (I didn't even have one). I was so nervous I thought the assistant was reading my mind and could tell that they were for me. I soon stopped worrying though, when you crave something all fear goes out of the window. I now think that my impulsive personality made me prone to addiction. At that moment in time it was laxatives and I was just pouring them down my throat, tub after tub. I have no idea how long I kept up this vicious cycle. What I do know is that with the combination of laxative abuse, vomiting and starvation the weight started dropping off me. I lost about three and a half stone, enough to cause problems. My periods never stopped which could have been due to the contraceptive pill I was on. I had real troubles trying to find clothes to fit, everything just hung off me. Ironically the control I had so desperately craved was now controlling me. The body I had obsessively desired was now hidden in baggy clothes. I only achieved the creation of another vicious cycle, this time affecting both my physical and mental health. I didn't know how to stop it.

After having seen me for a weekend, following a long sailing trip abroad, my sister Sue phoned me and said "Lorry you're anorexic. You need help". I actually thought am I? She's wrong I have not got a problem. Although my sister's diagnosis wasn't a medical one, my doctor classified me as having an eating disorder. The label list was beginning to grow. I did receive a great deal of help and support from my GP at my weekly 'weigh ins', also from my then, current boyfriend, a close male colleague and above all my family who gave me unconditional love.

I've been asked before how did you stop it? The answer is I really don't know. Maybe it was an increase in self-esteem, happiness, confidence and security. Or purely the fact that now everyone knew, it was too difficult to pursue these abnormal behaviours. Although eating disorders can be controlled I don't believe the memory of them ever completely leaves you. I can go for weeks weighing myself everyday, often twice a day to see if I've put on a pound. I feel pretty uncomfortable sitting in this hospital, as I've been unable to use a set of scales in three weeks. At times I feel comfortable with my curves, whilst on other days I can be obsessed with feeling and looking fat. I very rarely allow myself treats such as crisps, chocolates or cakes. However, it does seem to be closely related to my state of mind. When depressed I have no appetite and have to force myself to eat, but when I'm high I seem to be too fast and busy to have the time or need to eat. For me this illness is not something you can say 'never again' to. It stays with you haunting and challenging your resolves. An example of this is when I go out for a meal or simply just having food in the restaurant here. I can't bear to eat with strangers, just the act of putting food in my mouth in front of someone else repulses me and it takes all the effort in the world to do. Yet again alcohol rears its familiar face. My coping mechanism, my saviour is to have a few drinks, or to be more honest quite a few, before I sit down to a public meal. Being a 'recovering alcoholic' means that I no longer have this option available to me. What happens at the next social function? I can already begin to feel the waves rising again in the wind. These issues still need more thought, or more precisely thought changing. It seems to tentatively be under control, but I guess I'm still waiting for the sunrise.

CHAPTER FIVE – THE WILL TO STAY AFLOAT

Suicide! Can another person actually understand the unique personal emotions that an individual feels when contemplating suicide? I've read a lot of literature about this subject and in fairness have come across various people who 'live' up to it. The following explanations have often been put forward; A cry for help, wanting to teach others a lesson, wanting to show others how much you love them, stopping someone leaving you. The list could go on forever. I'm not here to judge anyone; again someone's own pain is true to them. I just know it felt differently for me.

I knew at the Social Club after work that I would take my own life that night. It had taken over my mind for weeks and seemed the only option. I needed to get out, to leave or to dissolve. I felt desperate. I was yet again extremely depressed with my mind, body and soul in absolute agony. I couldn't bear the anxiety and agitation. I was determined not to face another day again. All I desperately asked for, craved for, pleaded for, was peace of mind and to feel calm within myself. These two things are all I ever desire, but I so easily lose track of them when I'm sailing between the hypomanias and depression.

When I returned to the flat I made sure no one else was around and carried out my calculated suicide plan in a very calm manner. I'd had a few drinks earlier but wasn't drunk, I put my then favourite music on (Genesis I think) and I was wearing a T-shirt that Sue had given me (she was abroad again). The music was down low, as were the lights, I sat on my bed and took everything and anything I could lay my hands on (this included my prescribed antidepressants and tranquilizers). I then lay upon my bed, relaxed and peaceful, just waiting for release. Desperate yet quiet, feeling sure that this was the end of a very long nightmare. The only reasons, aims and desires for my suicide attempt were death. As simple as that, I wanted to die, I wanted an end.

The next thing I became aware of, was being bundled into a car by a group of friends. Apparently, my flat mate (a good friend at that point) had come home, noticed the low lights and music and decided to come in for a chat. Obviously, I hadn't put the music and lights on low enough. I'm not sure if she found me unconscious, but I was obviously aroused enough to be bundled into the car. Most of what follows is a drugged blur. I remember that a stomach washout was rather viciously attempted (the nurse concerned was reprimanded at a later date), but this failed. I was also admitted to a ward I had recently worked on, was put into a NHS nightdress and given a charcoal suspension to drink (which absorbs the drugs). The whole experience was humiliating and degrading. I just lay in my hospital bed thinking, "It didn't work", over and over again. I wanted to scream out in agony and pain.

The anger I felt towards my friends was huge. Why did they have to 'help', why hadn't they just left me alone? It was my decision. I had made it and had carried it through. How could anyone tear it away from me? Why was my freedom of choice taken away? I had so many unanswered questions. I now know that I wasn't well enough to make such decisions, but that wasn't how I viewed it at the time. I ended up seeing the duty Psychiatrist for five minutes, literally, in a box room, with NHS nightie on, charcoal around my face and a blanket around my shoulders. How could he miss that I was severely clinically depressed, even with the little knowledge I had, I knew there was something seriously wrong. I know I didn't want anything 'done', but that was because I wanted to be dead not alive. Surely it must be ethically wrong to ignore such desolation in a patient. Perhaps it was because I never left a suicide note. I didn't leave one purely because I had nothing to say, I just wanted out. So, I was psychologically patted on the head and sent on a week's leave to Portsmouth. After all, nothing more is needed to treat clinical depression (yes sarcasm - it happens).

The one person I need to mention here in a little more detail was my boyfriend at the time. On my discharge he took me by the hand and led me on a somewhat lengthy climb up a nearby hill. We lay on our backs looking at the moon and stars for what seemed like hours. I didn't need to give a detailed explanation, he knew, he understood, words were pointless. I think this is one man I actually fell in love with in Bath. He was my soul mate. We could spend hours talking about anything or listening to music (another great passion of mine) into the early hours of the morning. I guess there were a few rather large downfalls. His alcohol problem was greater then mine, we both had depressive natures and he was even more frightened of commitment than I was. We made two attempts at this relationship, but it fell apart when I moved back to Portsmouth to live. It was a case of we can't live together and can't live apart. I know I hurt him badly, I never meant to. It was just that our shared dream would never have been more than that, only a dream. Even now I can close my eyes and see his spontaneous smile and deep sparkling eyes. I will always think of him as an extremely special person.

The next major event was to phone my parents, to say, "Hi it's Lorry, how's your day been? Oh yes, I've just tried to kill myself." Mum, although very upset, wasn't surprised, she had been expecting something of this nature. My Dad was unable to talk to me, as he had absolutely no understanding. I spent a lot of time watching the waves break on the beach, trying to work out where my life was heading. There was talk of me joining Sue and Andy on a passage for the yacht they were working on. This didn't materialize so my parents watched me get back on the train to Bath, despite their reluctance and misgivings. Now having children of my own I can only envisage the pain, agony and distress they must have felt letting me go back into the unknown.

The problem or miracle was (and is) that I am an absolute fighter and won't give up until the end and even then I go down shouting and cursing. Maybe this has been my savior and that is why I am still here now. My only true best friend John met me at the train station, full of hugs, jokes and wise cracks. His strength and laughter kept me going so many times. It was so hard returning to work, there were so many stares and whispers behind doors. Somehow I held my head high knowing all the time that I was the latest newsbeat at the hospital.

The next saving grace was starting my placement at the Casualty Department within three weeks of my overdose. I decided to be brave and went to both the Sister and Charge Nurse to confess my recent sins. They were fantastic and mentioned that other members of staff within the department had been in similar situations to me. At first I couldn't even go into the room where I'd had my attempted stomach washout. I found it too emotionally painful. However, within a few weeks I was allocated all of the attempted suicide cases. I think it was because I could show genuine empathy and for some reason, I was extremely focused and had a clear positive attitude. Maybe it was because I was so happy working within this department. I was even able to kick my Lorazepam addiction with their support and I was never judged. Unsurprisingly, I thrived on the high intensity situations and would feel hugely satisfied delivering the psychological care that was constantly required.

I have always been the type of nurse that attempts to imagine what it would be like to be my patient. This has resulted in both emotional and unusual experiences. For example I have worn a stomach bag for 24 hours (filled with water), to help one of my patients accept their own colostomy. This proved to be beneficial to both of us as we were able to have a realistic and honest discussion. I've always built great rapport with my patients and their relatives and dedicated 100% effort to their care, no matter what mood state I would find myself in.

Before I delve into my second overdose in Bath, I need to discuss certain issues I had with men and relationships. I was promiscuous. I will freely admit that. If I examine that fact it could be for a number of reasons. How embarrassing, well here goes. Firstly, I think I was craving acceptance, love, affection, and respect...from a man. I'm sure this was due to the poor relationship with my dad. I think I only really wanted innocent love and companionship and this was the only way I thought I could get it. I would have short relationships or one night stands, occasionally not knowing their names. Afterwards I would hate myself and would think "you slut, tart, slag", but after all, these were only names I'd heard before, so what's new? When I felt depressed, being physically close to someone would lift my spirits, only a little, but enough to get some comfort. Another factor, again rearing its ugly head, was alcohol. Most nights I was drunk to varying degrees and we all know that alcohol reduces your inhibitions. I'm sure I had sex with a lot of men whom I wouldn't even have considered in sober circumstances. Finally and at the moment most significantly, was that many of the situations I found myself in could be due to the fact that I was indeed hypomanic. I obviously didn't understand why at that point, but I did go through cycles where I would be extremely promiscuous and become obsessed with sex. I would think that I was amazingly attractive and sexy, that I was extremely good in bed and every man would want me. No wonder I had very few close friends. On a superficial level it did mean that I was fun to go clubbing with and who cared what I did afterwards? I didn't at the time, so why should anyone else care?

The next event has only come up recently, hidden away in my subconscious memory. It's been suddenly catapulted to the surface at the cost of much distress. I don't know if my sexual antics had any persuasion on the situation. Maybe, but I think most probably not, as at a later date I discovered it had happened to a couple of other nurses. I had been working with a

Registrar for a number of weeks. He was the type that was full of chat, sexual innuendos and comments. Above all he was a creep, he made me feel extremely uncomfortable and very wary. The comments had been going on for weeks, such as "we should get together, have a good time, you'd enjoy it", etc, etc. I always point blank refused. This must say something in itself, considering the state I was in.

One evening I went to the Social Club for an after work pint, a habit established by most nurses. I was feeling low and ended up talking to this man. More foolishly I let him buy me a second pint, something I had never done before. You need to be aware that during those days I could easily drink 7 pints and still find my own way home, comfortably. I remember drinking the first half but that is it.

The next thing I knew I was feeling groggy and heady. It was daylight, obviously early morning and I was lying in a stranger's bed completely naked, with my clothes strewn across the floor. I looked around and there was this creep with a smarmy grin on his face, as though to say 'I told you I would'. The expression 'the bottom fell out of my world' was extremely suited. I felt confused and disorientated. I couldn't remember anything apart from the fact that I'd had hardly anything to drink. The first and only words spoken were his. "Don't worry I used condoms on you". At this moment my fears were confirmed, I jumped up, got dressed and ran home straight into a hot shower. I felt shocked, for a number of reasons. I'd not been a saint, but surely I didn't deserve this, or did I? After all, I was a worthless slut, tart, slag, whore and this just confirmed it. Having to continue working with this man was a waking nightmare, but I did and I kept my mouth shut, which I'm sure he knew I would. So for all these years I have kept this blocked, shut away in a box until recently. What amaze me are the feelings of disgust, dirt, filth, fear and hate. They are as real now as they were then.

The final part of this chapter, if you can actually believe it, seems even worse because I wasn't drugged this time. After my Casualty placement my soul mate and I went to Turkey for a 2 week, backpacking holiday. I think, on reflection, my moods were quickly flying between highs and lows so I may have been experiencing a mixed state. My boyfriend loved it when I was high, at these times we got on really well. However, when I was low he threatened to leave and continue the holiday alone. I know he must have been confused but not half as much as I was. I thought sod it, if he's going to walk off I'll just get on with it. On return to England our relationship finished for the first time. After a while of playing around I met Ernie, a man who I thought (not realizing the dangers) appeared loving, caring, kind and considerate. He really pushed the boat out; wined me, dined me, flowers, the whole works. I remained wary, unsurprisingly, and kept my distance.

The next thing I knew, he was admitted at my hospital, under the false pretences of having appendicitis. This was purely to find out which ward I worked on, where he came to visit me and freely admitted the whole scam. At this point little alarm bells started to ring. We continued the relationship and the 'prince' turned into a 'monster from the deep'! I was an easy victim at that point with low self- esteem, suffering with depression and feeling worthless. I did manage to keep some of my faculties though, I realized he was bad news and tried to get out of the relationship. We were in a public place and he could only just contain his rage. When he took me home he attacked me verbally. " You're a complete head case, you shouldn't be alive, you need a shrink and you are a waste of space!". After about an hour of this abuse (I couldn't physically make him go, he was a big man!) I was left alone, believing all that he had said to me. To start with, I was extremely fragile and depressed, now I was a complete wreck and he knew it.

I needed to sleep so I took some sedatives, but then I just didn't stop. Not until every drug in my room had been swallowed. Although to start with I just wanted to sleep, my obsessive suicidal thoughts crept in, until they were screaming at me. Again I think my impulsive nature took over and once I started I couldn't stop. I think I was most probably unconscious for the rest of the night (I had taken the pills quite early), but somehow I roused myself for work. Once I got there I was obviously far too drugged to be safe and was very ill. I made my excuses and went home to my room. The next 48 hours I'd imagine, were the closest a living person could get to a walk through hell. Between bouts of unconsciousness, I hallucinated like nothing on earth. I guess I certainly know now what a drug induced 'trip' is. I had bouts of diarrhoea and vomiting, with just a sink in my room. I couldn't risk using the communal toilet and in reality I wouldn't have physically made it there. Trying to clear up in that state was a near impossible task.

So why didn't I ask for help? I didn't want to. I was depressed and the remains of my being had been destroyed. My thoughts were: 'great, let me die. I've no problems with that. Just let me go now. I deserve it. I've taken the risk so I have to go through with it. I'm not worthy to live anyway'. The Staff Nurse from my placement had guessed something was wrong so he sent his girlfriend round to help. I couldn't/wouldn't let her in; instead I just shouted through the door that I was fine. So there I was, sat waiting for release from this vicious squall. The most terrifying part was the hallucinations, two of which still remain vivid in my memory.

Firstly, I could see men hanging from the curtain rail. Their eyes were bulging and their tongues swollen, forcibly hanging from their mouths. The men's bodies were swollen and misshapen, as if damaged and there were flies all around them. In spite of my drugged mind I was desperately trying to reach them to help, however the gap between us never decreased. The bodies just kept swaying backwards and forwards in an unconnected breeze. In this hallucination I was actually convinced it was happening, however in the second one I was painfully aware that I was hallucinating. In the past, I had observed many confused, elderly patients carry out the following behaviour: they would be sitting quietly, concentrating meticulously, all their efforts aimed at plucking invisible objects out of the air in front of them. I sat on my bed doing exactly that, driven by some invisible force, to pluck those transparent objects from out of the air in front of me. I thought 'shit Lorry you're hallucinating', but I carried on regardless, I just couldn't bring myself to stop. I do feel angry at these moments, if I had received proper psychiatric care much earlier, then it may have saved me from this experience. About 48 hours after I overdosed I went to my GP. He was horrified that I had told no one and wanted to admit me there and then. My therapist stopped him with the argument that if he took my work away from me, I would have no aims or goals and that I would lose my fighting spirit. Somewhat reluctantly my GP decided that my care would remain community-based. Was the therapist right or wrong? I don't know. Another case of what if, I guess.

The next occurrence was that Ernie, the bullying creep, appeared yet again out of nowhere. By then I was completely deflated and confused about everything. His natural domination just took over and I entered a realm of physical, mental and sexual abuse. I found myself completely ensnared in a life of paralyzing fear. He was so scheming and crafty. The bruises never showed, or they could be easily explained away. The mental anguish that he inflicted upon me was quietly transmitted, not for others to hear. Just continual attacks: e.g. "it's your fault, your guilty, your worthless, no-one will ever want you". It felt like brain washing and in fact, was very effective. The worst part was the sexual abuse and it is obviously the hardest part to write about. If we refer back to the sailing, I was in the worst raging storm ever, with a central whirlwind pulling me in deeper. My self-esteem was reduced to zero through the constant comparisons that he made to his previous conquests. These could have been lies or actually descriptions of others anguish. That man abused me, degraded me, made me feel like a slab of meat and forced me to perform the most painful and disgusting acts ever. I would beg, cry and plead for him to stop, starting with a shout, reducing to a whisper and then finally into a beaten murmur. Yet again I was left feeling humiliated, dirty and violated. This was not a one off situation, it was repeated time and again. I had not been drugged this time to dim the emotional and physical pain.

As I write this I just want to sit and cry, let the tears ebb out, but I'm scared the tide will never flow back in again. This violent relationship continued, purely as a result of my own fear and terror. Do not judge others in a similar situation, as fear can be all encompassing. We ended up getting engaged, as a result of my trying to leave him. Ernie had exhibited more dominating control and had threatened to kill me if I did leave, hence the engagement. At a later date on speaking to his ex wife, I discovered that she had tried to get warnings through to me, only to be blocked every time by Ernie. My parents were suspicious of him, so the best support they could offer was to let him move in with them in Portsmouth, until I returned from Bath. This way they felt they could at least keep an eye on the situation.

Finally, once he'd left Bath I plucked up the courage to tell Sue what was really going on and this enabled me to be strong enough to write to him and finish the relationship. Guess what? He travelled from Portsmouth and turned up on my doorstep. I wasn't going to get away with it that easily. He made so much noise that I had to let him into the flat. Boy he was in a rage, the noise and violence was so great that my flat mates were too scared to leave their rooms, apart from one friend and I was so frightened for her safety that I shouted at her to go away. Imagine my terror, as I was alone in the same room as him. After a lot of violence I resorted to trying to strangle him in self-defence, but he was such a big man. I may as well have just put my arm around him for all the effect it had. This may be a bad thing to admit, but I can clearly see how at times in domestic violence, an individual can end up grabbing a knife and using it in self-defence. By the morning he said that he was going to the Casualty Department, to tell them that one of their nurses had attacked him. Thankfully, I was both strong and drained enough to say: "fine go ahead and do it", at that point I was past caring.

I was still terrified of him at our final meeting. He had moved out of my parents' home and was working in a hotel where he rented a room. He insisted that I met him alone in his room; Sue came with me and waited in the car. I remained determined and met him in the very busy, public entrance. Ernie had a fixed smile on his face for show, but through those gritted teeth he promised to kill me the next time he saw me. He still owes my parents money, but they aren't worried, they'd rather I'm blessed with never seeing him again. They take comfort in knowing that he's out of my life for good. The thought of coming face to face with him still fills me with terror to this day.

So that was Bath. When I sit here and read through this, it amazes me that so many dreadful things could happen to an individual, in such a short space of time. The pain, fear and hurt are still there but I have to live with it. Mostly the memories are in the past where they belong, but at times they are very much in the present, along with the nightmares of course. Maybe it was the wrong approach, but all I could do at the time was acknowledge those feelings and move on and that is exactly what I did. I had to work out my sick time and I consequently qualified later then the rest of my group. On completion I returned to Portsmouth as a Registered General Nurse, an outstanding accomplishment all things considered!

CHAPTER SIX – THE HUM OF THE HULL

In comparison the next three years were a breeze, but not completely without my mood swings or certain events. On return to Portsmouth, I moved back in with my parents for a limited amount of time and I financially supported myself with agency work. As soon as I could afford to, I bought my own car and moved into a shared 'professional' (I could finally call myself one) house. The plan was to go and work in Romania as nurses with my 'soul' mate. However, in my wisdom I was talked into a careers interview, with an aim to enter the world of counselling. During the interview I was informed that a degree in psychology would be more appropriate to my qualifications and would give me greater scope. Before I realized it, I was having an informal chat with my former psychology lecturer. He fully agreed and contacted his colleague at the head of psychology admissions at Portsmouth University. Once started in motion the wheels kept turning and I was suddenly heading on my way down to the university.

The journey (all of 5 miles) to my 'interview' was not without complications! I heard a strange noise whilst driving and as I was in a hurry I just turned the radio up. Much flashing later by my fellow motorists, found me at a garage with a flat tyre, an hour and a half late and covered in oil, grime and grease. What a great first impression this would be! On top of that I was so nervous at meeting this wonderful gentleman, I knocked my coffee all over his desk!! Thank goodness it was yet again an informal chat and not an interview in front of a board of lecturers.

For me, this was both amazing and fantastic; I now had a place at University reading a Bachelor of Science Honours Degree in Psychology, which would commence in a few weeks time. What a career interview that turned out to be, it certainly opened some doors! Suddenly it hit me, big time. Was I actually good enough to be doing this? Did I have the brains to do this? After all, I wasn't the intelligent one; my sister was instead I was the blonde bimbo. How was I going to financially support myself? This was a big commitment. Unsurprisingly, I received a lot of opposition, some genuine and others silly concerns. I need to acknowledge one friend who fuelled and encouraged my determination throughout this period. An unpleasant action that I had to take was to tell my boyfriend from Bath that I would not be going to Romania as discussed. I always knew these were just dreams that couldn't compete with the alcohol. None the less, it was a hard blow and we have not stayed in touch. I would like to see him again, just once to explain. I guess that will never happen.

Over the summer I had pretty constant agency work at a private hospital so I joined their bank staff. This is how I independently financed myself throughout the three years of my degree, an accomplishment I'm very proud of. I would quite often do a night shift followed by course work during my breaks and then in the mornings go straight into university for lectures. I wonder if I was actually going through manic phases at these times, as I was indestructible. My first day at university, sitting in the lecture auditorium, was one of the proudest in my life even in comparison to graduation day. I just couldn't quite believe that I was sitting there, that it wasn't a joke and that I'd soon be asked to move along. I was actually intelligent enough to belong there. This was so huge because it was always presumed that I wasn't clever enough, so I never imagined I could do it.

Whilst I was living in the professional house, I didn't have one-night stands, but yet again I had a wide range of boyfriends with maybe the same reasons as before. Two of the most important things that happened to me whilst I was living here were: firstly I was introduced to the wonders of large yacht sailing and secondly I got to know my sister's friend Andy a lot better. I ended up moving house (as per usual) numerous times, until I was semi settled with a girlfriend in a 2 up 2 down, centred in student land. I was living quite a bizarre life style. During the week I spent my time studying (enough to get by on), working to finance myself and eating baked beans on toast. Whilst at weekends I was sailing, nibbling on canapés and sipping champagne! I did have an initial consultation with a psychiatrist on my return to Portsmouth and although I didn't need a follow up, he informed me that the service's doors were always open to me. I also saw a cognitive psychologist for about eighteen months, which helped me greatly as I seemed to be able to relate to cognitive therapy very well.

I need to talk about my sailing now, to enable you to grasp some understanding of what it means to me. There were three types really: the racing and partying scene, the working with guest's scene and the passaging or general sailing. For once I fitted into all of the above categories. Again, I now know that when I combined the working, racing and partying scenes (as I frequently did) I was most probably high. However, when I was passaging (on a journey) or just simply sailing I really believe that I was actually myself, just Lorry. Not Lorry with an illness or being high or low, but just Lorry. At this point it was the only time that I had been myself and it felt fantastic.

My most wonderful calm, peaceful and happy times in the world were the night watches. These were spent sometimes alone and sometimes with others. Holding onto the wheel with the rush of water racing under the hull, causing it to occasionally hum. With the sails full of wind forcing us along with such power and feeling the vibration of speed through the wheel. This was magical, but you really need to be there to experience the sensation. I don't think my words could ever do it justice. A fantastic bonus to this was the night sky inky and vast, the stars sparkling like nothing else on this planet. Of course there would be times when it was cloudy, cold, stormy, windy and raining; but I loved all the elements, it was just a different challenge as far as I could see. It would make me feel alive. A further experience, which would leave me speechless night or day, would be adding playful dolphins to the moment. I would be transfixed whilst they played in the bow waves, speaking to one another. They were simply and purely happy. For someone who suffers with mental illness that is an astonishing sight to witness, sheer happiness just 'because' and I absorbed it.

The next phase was a riot, still immensely fun, but I dare say I was high during these long periods usually over a summer. The owner of the yacht was a wonderful city businessman, extremely generous and I thought the world of him. My main racing was out of the Hamble and Cowes, but I also sailed in regattas at Cork, Guernsey and St Tropez. My longest passage on this yacht was from the Hamble, to Spain (across the Bay of Biscay), on to Gibraltar, Minorca and then finally to the south of France.

Basically, during racing periods, there would be long days of hard physical labour, long nights of partying and drinking and countless people to get to know (yet again that promiscuous high of mine would step in). One experience that makes me laugh (now!) took place at Cork in Ireland. It was an extremely windy day and I slipped on the foredeck, I landed on a large cleat. I struggled on for a couple of days, racing but barely able to walk. I eventually submitted to seeing the doctor. I had fractured my coccyx (tail bone) and I had to use a blown up life jacket to sit on. Consequently, my homeward travel arrangements were changed and I had to fly home instead. When I walked down the aisle (we were nearly the first to board) I think everyone turned white with fear. The other passengers saw what they thought was a healthy person, walk onto the plane with a blown up life jacket! Their faces said it all, 'what do you know that we don't?'

The working and chartering part was extremely hard work. I'd committed myself to Andy that summer as his hostess/first mate, so in spite of the fractured coccyx I still worked for him. My job consisted of ensuring that the boat was spotless, preparing and serving food (gourmet cooking), helping Andy sail the yacht, entertaining guests (albeit at times frustrating) and meticulously cleaning up afterwards. It was hard work and due to the fracture painful, but fun and after all I was out sailing everyday which beat working in a hospital!

During that summer Sue and Andy were having problems with their relationship. Sue had met her present husband (a lovely person) and Andy turned to me for comfort and support. We often shared a bottle of wine (or two) after work and got on extremely well together. I also started working on a larger yacht, as cook/hostess, passaging up to Wales and Scotland with four men. Now THIS was bloody hard work. They all behaved like male chauvinists and as though they didn't have a female on board. However we had great fun, loads of laughs and drinking and I adored them all. I know the feeling was mutual and they all complained that they'd put on too much weight due to my cooking! Our first night was quite amusing, you need to keep in mind that I didn't know any of these guys at all. I didn't do watches, as I had to make their breakfasts etc. I was fast asleep in one of the top bunks, before I was properly awake I realized that Nick, the youngest guy whom I shared a cabin with, was fumbling around in my bunk, with me still in it! I jumped up rather shocked, until I realized he was sleep walking! As I was now awake, I went up on deck for a fag and a cup of tea and I joked with the rest of the crew as to what had just happened. I returned to sleep and a little later, while Nick, oblivious to all, awoke to the others' story that he had touched me up, that I was absolutely disgusted and I would be jumping ship in the morning. The look on his face at breakfast was a picture and I wasn't even aware of any of the false claims they had told him! It was soon resolved with a lot of laughter.

Very sadly this part of my book has an extremely tragic end and I still find it hard to believe even now. After the summer season, arrangements were in motion for the yacht to go to the Caribbean with Nick and Jon (two of the guys I had just worked with). I was offered a chance to go with them and grabbed it with both hands. However, it wasn't until later deliberation and soul searching, that I realized I wouldn't actually return to my degree as I had promised myself. With many regrets I decided not to go with them. Devastatingly, once in the Caribbean, the yacht and therefore the innocent people on board, were horrifically mistaken as being involved in a drugs deal. Jon, Nick and two guests on board were tortured and murdered. How can this be? It just doesn't happen to real, normal, everyday people. They were individuals that had so much to live for and so much ahead of them. It's like a section from a Hollywood film, not something that has really happened to two of my sailing buddies. I guess you can tell that I still can't believe it happened, even ten years later. It may appear clichéd, but it only seems like yesterday that we were all sitting up on deck laughing over a mug of tea. Such a pointless loss, I dedicated my dissertation to Nick and Jon and I hope they have found some sea to sail on wherever they may be. It wasn't until later that the realization hit me; I could have been with them.

On return from Scotland I joined Andy and a few others for the passage down to the south of France. It was a wonderful experience and will always hold great memories for me. On arrival, the crew left, while Andy and I prepared the boat for our first guests. It was fantastic in St Tropez and visiting all the other elite marinas along the coast. I don't think I had ever partied properly before my experiences in this port. It was continual drinking and dancing until 4a.m. and then we would have to be up at 6a.m. to prepare breakfast for the guests and organize their daily entertainment and lunches. It was great and I belonged, after all I was a real 'yachty' now!

After this hectic time the Niolargue race week commenced which was fantastic fun. It consisted of hard competitive racing during the day, with meals out and serious socializing by night. I guess by now that it was pretty obvious that I had entered another manic state, along with my recurring promiscuous ways. However, my behaviours and attitudes were not amiss here, maybe everybody had a touch of mania! Or more likely it was just a case of my behaviour being within an acceptable context. Whilst we were there Andy confessed that he was falling in love with me. I don't think I was surprised, but I was confused, after all Andy was my big brother substitute and it just didn't feel right. As you can imagine during this whole period ashore, alcohol became a big part of my life again.

At the end of the regatta I flew back to England as my second year at university had started. Andy sailed back and it seemed an awful long time without him. Once home I discovered that Sue had started a relationship with her male friend, I felt so confused and upset. The two people that meant the most to me, the two people that had always been there for me, had just turned my world upside down. I guess it was a wake up call and a realization that even strong or established love doesn't always last forever. The next six months were hard as it always is in a long-term relationship break-up. Andy was convinced that he loved me and I really wanted to love him back. I knew I loved him on a certain level, but no matter how hard I tried, it could only be platonic. A bit ironic for me, as this was the one time I really wanted a physical relationship, yet I couldn't. Occasionally, I have wondered what if, but then what will be will be.

Another of my great sailing accomplishments was at the following year's Niolargue race week. Originally, my lecturer had refused me the time off to take part in it, as it meant that I would have to miss a week of term time in my final year. Not perturbed by this, I decided I would conduct my dissertation in St Tropez during the Niolargue race week, thus keeping my lecturer happy and me sailing! After completing a comprehensive and detailed research, I decided to compare different leadership styles of the skippers, both their own perceptions and that of their crews, with the different yachts' racing performances. My paper received a great deal of interest, both of a psychological nature and from a yachting perspective. Although I'd started off just wanting a weeks sailing I put an awful lot of work into my dissertation, even gaining knowledge from one of my patients who specialised in management skills. This hard work was reflected by the results and the enthusiasm shown by my lecturer in a bid to get me to publish it!

Somewhere amongst these latter experiences I met my husband. It was meant to be a one-night stand and yet again we didn't know each other's names. The love wasn't suddenly there over night; instead it was slow and gradual, happening along the way. We moved in together, Dan went off to sea and I sat my finals. At first it was hard being in a relationship where there was no physical presence of your partner or contact with them for months on end. To be honest, it has only really taken me until now to deal with it. As he is a submariner, he is away on these terms for a large proportion of the year. After our engagement we decided to set the wedding date for within 3 months, this certainly made the parents flap. Our wedding was a great party, with loads of alcohol (no surprise yet again) and lots of fun. Just before our wedding was another very important day for me, my graduation. I felt extremely proud, even more so because my dad (no doubts on my brains now), my mum and Dan were there to watch me. I must admit I did look rather strange in my graduation outfit and I can't bare the official photo, purely because I look drunk, as not surprisingly I was. In the evening a large gathering of my immediate family joined us to celebrate over a meal and some wine.

Once things had returned to normal and we were back from a great honeymoon, Dan disappeared back to sea and I started a full time contract job at the private hospital. This was my first 'proper' job since I had qualified as a nurse. To celebrate Dan bought me a silver nurse's belt buckle, in the shape of a dolphin (of course!). However, another tempting offer was on the horizon. Sue was taking time off from her job to sail across the Pacific Ocean with some old friends. Just before Christmas it evolved that they were short of crew and there was space for me, would I go? So five months later, nearly to the day of our wedding, I jumped (well shook violently!) on the first of many planes heading for Panama.

CHAPTER SEVEN – A PASSAGE TO PARADISE

I think I would have to describe this journey as a passage of challenges and wonderment. To enable me to write this chapter I've reread my travel journal and it was definitely not all bliss. Again, I will take an honest approach and convey to you best I can, this passage of a lifetime. The journey to Panama City took 33 hours with 8 take offs and landings. This isn't bad going, considering that before I left I was scared of flying, let alone doing it solo. On arrival I handed over all my documents to my contact, a man called Richard. Through my jet-lagged mind I was thinking 'I don't even know this man!' Again, I don't want to give a chronological documentation of events, it would take too long, instead I want to write from my heart on different experiences.

Brad and Ann, the yacht owners', were a retired American couple fulfilling his dream of sailing around the world. After 'night watch analysis' (we would discuss everything in detail during our watch) Sue and I decided that Ann didn't actually want to be there and was only doing it for Brad's pleasure. That was all very noble, but you need a lot more than that to keep you sailing around the world. I certainly wouldn't attempt it for the love of someone else. I'm not dismissing love, but a person has to live with hardships, isolation and even danger on a daily basis. I think ultimately you need a genuine love of the sea and sailing to keep you persevering through the hard times. A global racing sailor we know has said that he would like to sail the Whitbread Challenge with Sue and I as we have such quiet determination and resolve, two traits that are greatly needed apparently!

Ann seemed to have a big problem with me, as it soon became apparent that I was to be her scapegoat for a whole range of things. Sue was her favourite and she would let everyone know it. Brad when alongside was more relaxed and fun, however when at sea he became lazy, demanding and sexist. One of the more tense times would be the build up to starting a passage, it was a nightmare and the atmosphere could have been cut with a knife. I wonder what they say about us!

However, there were still fantastic times. We travelled through the Panama Canal, a completely awesome experience, although our pilot was more interested in Sue's broken bikini; which was rather scary as he was meant to be keeping us safe! We felt so small in our forty-eight foot yacht compared to these huge tankers and cargo vessels, which were crammed alongside each other in the canal. As the water drained away everything towered above us like a super high-rise block of flats. Then we sailed onto Tobago Bay and the Las Perlas Islands. At the latter location we were listening to the radio when we heard a distress call, about one hundred miles away. Convicts had boarded the woman's yacht, her husband had been shot in the head and the intruders had escaped. Many yachts in the close proximity responded, whilst it brought home to us that piracy was a reality and no longer just fictitious characters in a children's story. We did have our own false alarm at a later date and I will explain shortly the fortunate misunderstanding that was made. From here we did the week's passage to The Galapagos islands. After a stay there, a three-week passage to the Marquasas Islands followed (for which I will try to find some words to illustrate this magical place) and then my epic journey home.

One of the main reasons for undertaking this trip was my love of marine life (and of course the sailing!). Just snorkelling opened up a completely new world, or even watching the graceful sea birds. My main aim was to be able to observe whales in their natural habitat. However, they always seemed to be somewhere else and I would imagine this was due to the large number of factory ships we saw. I described in my travel journal one unexpected encounter we had with a whale shark at the Las Perlas Islands: 'well, the main thing that happened today was the 'shark attack'. Sue and I were rubbing the wood down on the boat whilst in the dinghy and Sue shouted "get out Lorraine, get out of the dinghy!" I looked around and saw this massive whale shark, twice the size of the dinghy and I just hung onto the guardrail. When we were up on the bow, we looked down and saw it slowly go pass the dinghy then across the bow. I was shaking!' We weren't at risk as whale sharks are harmless, I think it was more the sheer size and close proximity of the shark that alarmed us.

The Galapagos are a set of volcanic islands, which have unique wildlife and this is where the naturalist Darwin carried out a vast majority of revolutionary work. Again, I am concentrating on the emotional aspect of this experience, so if you have a desire for more facts, you'll have to research them yourself! Anyway, Sue and I joined a group of young people (fantastic!) hiring a motorboat and crew to take us around some of the islands for a few days.

This had to be done with an official guide, so it got rather costly. As we were on a budget luxury was removed from the price, which afforded us no comfort, no privacy, no pleasant smells and no cleanliness. What the hell - the food was good!

We visited a number of islands and although the scenery was out of this world, it was the truly spectacular wildlife that stole the show for me. Snorkelling with the sea lions was amazing; they quite literally played with you. Racing in and out, chasing us around, whilst stopping their faces a few centimetres from our masks. However, we had to give the bulls a wide birth as they were extremely protective and could be very aggressive. We also swam with penguins, white tipped sharks, turtles and fish of every colour imaginable. The penguins and turtles were so graceful underwater and the vision of them took my breath away. The turtles glided with what appeared to be no effort, sailing through the water; whilst the penguins darted in and out of sight, like mini torpedoes. On shore we came face to face with iguanas (and a species that swam), Blue-Footed Boobies (they were literally bright blue), Masked Boobies, Frigate birds, finches and giant tortoises. We had to actually step over the Boobies so that we didn't tread on them. One of the most spiritual moments for me was the experience of the dark mangroves. It was so peaceful there, nothing moved (unless the occasional ray surfaced), not even the water, which was deep and dark but not foreboding. It's hard to describe what my feelings were, but I will try. It was as though I was at one with myself; submerged in complete calm, peace and tranquility. Maybe I found part of the true Lorry here as well.

Finally, as we were leaving, we passed by an active volcanic island and this was a magnificent sight, although our photos didn't do it justice. It was as though the surrounding seascape had been transformed into a Turkish steam bath as the molten lava hit the water and disappeared into a fog of steam. I wrote my final thoughts of the Galapagos Islands in my travel journal: 'The Galapagos are an exquisite place and has or will have alone, made this three and a half month journey worth it.... These 4 days have been a unique chance in a lifetime, which I have loved. I've quite possibly been in heaven on earth. My deepest regret is that Dan isn't here to experience these spiritually, enchanted islands with me'.

This introduces me to the next topic, how desperately I missed Dan, to the extent that I flew home a few weeks early. I don't think I would have done now, but life is different when you're younger, especially as a newly married couple. I can remember sitting and talking with Sue, saying that in a few years time and with our children running around, I'll be able to sit in my comfy chair and say "yes I did that, no regrets". It was bloody hard and tested me to the limits, but sitting here albeit in a comfy, hospital chair, I can sit and say, "Yes I did it and no regrets". It's amazing how some bad experiences can fade with time. I found the three-week passage, especially with Brad and Ann, very difficult. I think my first mental block was that I didn't feel safe with them and for once in my life I had a fear of dying. In the past, no matter whom I sailed with, I always had great confidence and trust in the skipper and crew. I believed 100% in Sue and I, but not in Brad and Ann, at times they even frightened me. Also this was the longest passage with no landfall (3 weeks) I had ever done in the widest expanse of sea. So this time the 'survival at sea' briefs were for real. We even put together our own personal emergency packs to go in the life raft, just in case.

I was also missing Dan so much that it hurt. I really ached for him and I would often think that we'd only just got married; he was shore-based in Portsmouth for once so I would wonder what I was doing there. Sue and I also had our moments; it was quite a small space for 4 adults to live, especially as I love my own time so much. For instance, I obviously couldn't just go out for a walk, or pop off down to the shops. We had to re-establish roles i.e. the big/little sister relationship. However, we always solved our differences and it really did bring us closer together, a bond that will never be broken. This next extract out of my journal should, to a degree, illustrate how mind blowing it was: 'At times I feel as though we're not even moving. It seems as though someone had anchored us to the bottom and they have created an illusion that the sea is just flowing past us. It's amazing how vast this ocean is, with little alteration to the scenery apart from the waves and clouds. I feel as though I've been captured in a time warp or a void, as though nothing else existed, or exits now. It's pretty mind blowing, just the sea, sky, Brad, Ann and Sue.'

We didn't see any whales, much to my disappointment, I'm sure they were there, but just not wanting to be seen. I must also mention the night sky: I found it fantastic in Europe but now it was amazing, inspiring and literally out of this world. As there were no lights or pollution to obscure the sky above, we could see millions of stars nestling amongst the planets. I was in awe as Sue taught me many of their names. The only truly, frightening moment we experienced on the passage was the mistaking of fishermen to be pirates. We went for days with no shipping in sight and then suddenly there was this small boat heading straight for us. Sue and I quickly tried to disguise ourselves as men (I couldn't find anywhere to hide my boobs though!) and under Dick's breathe, we could hear him chanting to us all to "stay calm, stay calm" whilst none of us could imagine what terrors were about to befall us. We must have been frozen like that for a few minutes, when at the last moment they must have seen us and altered course, at which point we saw their fishing nets. We couldn't believe it: in all this space, in all this ocean, and we were nearly run down by a fishing vessel that never even saw us! It's funny now, but not then, not in those few minutes and not after the experience in Las Perlas. It certainly makes you realize how completely isolated and alone you are out there on that ocean.

The first thing that stunned me, as we approached the Marquesas Islands, was the lushness of the greenery. These islands were volcanic and every spare inch was covered with vegetation including wild mango, coco, pamplemousse and banana trees. We were soon joined by our other passaging comrades: the 'children' (i.e. younger adults) and 'parents' (i.e. older adults), as we were now fondly (?) called in our groups. It's bizarre really as nobody stopped talking; yet all we had to share was what we hadn't been doing and what we hadn't seen! Most probably we all just found it great to have some different and refreshing company. In my journal I have described these islands as beautiful, tranquil, spectacular and as one of the most spiritual places I have ever visited and even possibly in the world. These islands evoked the same emotions in me that the mangroves had in the Galapagos. There are just not enough words to describe such a wondrous place and I felt extremely privileged, as very few people get to see them.

One place that remains in the forefront of my mind was the local cemetery, this is what I wrote in my journal: 'On the Tuesday we did hand washing ashore and then had a group walk up to the local cemetery. It was beautiful, I walked alone as it was the only way to appreciate the tranquility, away from the others. The others found two famous graves, that of a French artist and another of a musician. The most stunning part for me was the view as it was breath taking. The monument that really took my breathe away was a statue of Jesus Christ on a crucifix, not only was it massive but also spectacular. This is saying something for me considering I'm not religious, I was almost but not quite tempted into believing, however I was moved enough into recognizing it was one of the most spiritual places I'd ever been to.'

After much discussion, thought and an awful lot of organization, I left these magical islands and although a few weeks early, I headed for home. I was scared to travel all that way alone, with two overnight stops, but I was determined and after all it was just another challenge. I had to take a helicopter to the other side of the island, this was an amazing flight and gave me a bird's eye view of the scenery and on landing I boarded a plane to Tahiti. Once there I caught a taxi across town and stayed in a youth hostel with mixed rooms, unfortunately the guy in the bunk above me seemed to forget he wasn't alone, rather an unusual experience in all! From here I flew to Los Angeles with a male traveling companion I had met at the Tahiti hostel. The place we stayed at couldn't be described as a hostel; it was grimy, dirty, run down and full of very dubious characters. My friend and I were offered a double bed that we hastily turned down, explaining we were only friends not partners. I was then offered a mattress in the women's room, and he in the men's. This made us both laugh; as on that basis we should have shared the bed after all, as he was gay! After having an agonising wait at the 'hostel', as I was reliant on them for transport, I managed to get on my flight home with just minutes to spare. Finally, I managed to get some sleep, the first since the Marquises Islands and I stepped off the plane in London into the long awaited arms of my husband. In all and in my armchair, this was a fabulous experience and I'm so glad I met the challenge.

There is one person I would like to mention and that is Sam. We spent time with him during the first part of our journey. He was from America and was spending five years sailing the world's oceans, researching dolphins whilst simultaneously getting close to and observing whales. This guy gave me (and Sue) so much strength, courage and peace. He was extremely spiritual and had an amazing aura and is someone I will never forget. On our goodbyes I gave him the book called 'Tao of Pooh', it holds such great thoughts and directions, which reminded me of him. I wonder if he still has it?

Rereading this I've realized how alcohol and partying played a really small role, whilst sex was redundant. I know I got extremely low at times and maybe verged on having depression, but on the whole I think I was reasonably stable, which is a comforting thought. This passage enabled me to find my inner strengths, learn about myself: as in who I am, what my beliefs were and what I was prepared to accept out of life and other people. Unfortunately, so much has happened since then that this no longer seems as realistic. Due to what has taken place in my life my expectations fail to be as certain, I can't even look as far as a month ahead, because at this moment I could easily be depressed or manic in the near future. Again and maybe through the writing of this book, I'm trying to discover who I really am as I've lost sight of the essence that has created me. However, I try to remember that there will always be a sunrise. There is always hope in a new day with the real belief that things are able to improve.

CHAPTER EIGHT – THE DEPRESSION AFTER THE HIGH

Before I'd left the UK our naval posting was for Faslane on the west coast of Scotland. Whilst in the Maquesas Islands, Dan however, informed me that we had moved to Bushey near Watford. Great I thought at least I didn't have to do any of the packing. When I finally arrived in our new home, I found strange goings on, such as shoes in laundry baskets and a BBQ in the wardrobe, so it looked as though I would have to do the unpacking after all. When I reached home I was greeted with champagne, roses and a romantic meal for two. It was heaven and I finally enjoyed something I hadn't been able to experience for months, a bath! We had discussed our options before I went away and reconfirmed them on the drive home. This was our plan: I would now try to get a psychology position in the city whilst we also tried for a baby. We had expected the latter to take months, how wrong could we be? I fell pregnant straight away and although it was a shock it was a good one. I then applied to the local private hospital and started bank work there. My pregnancy wasn't great; I was plagued with 'all day' morning sickness and had a few minor heart problems. Yet again though, the depression reared its ugly head and I suffered with it for most of the time. In conclusion to this, the birth was a living nightmare, which I don't cherish delving into now.

We started off at home, but the labour wasn't progressing, so we had to go into hospital with the midwife. Once there, I had an intravenous drip set up of

Syntocinin and I opted out of an epidural. One of my tranquil images I used to get through the pain was the memory of dolphins jumping through the bow waves on a crystal clear morning and it really did help. Everything started to go wrong when the midwife's shift ended and she was replaced. The main crunch was when I needed to remove my nightshirt. The new midwife should have switched the drip off when she removed it from the electronic infusion pump, but she didn't. The consequence of this non-action was that the majority of a litre bag of the drug syntocinin poured straight into me. I can remember thinking 'shit!' she hasn't switched it off, but I just wasn't physically capable of shouting out. From then on, it was a living hell. This sudden influx of syntocinin caused continual contractions and it was as though my whole body was possessed and convulsing. Then I had to have an epidural put in, but again due to the drug overdose, this wasn't straightforward. As my body was in continual spasms I ended up with a dural tap. This is when the membranes around the spinal column are nicked and the spinal fluid leaks out. Hence this resulted in extreme mind blowing headaches which hit a while afterwards and caused me to have two further admissions over the following few days. The midwife also left me sitting on metal bars, due to the epidural I no longer had movement from the waist down, which is not a great idea for someone with a coccyx injury. The room was a mess and really was just a reflection of the chaos we had to endure. At this point Dan left the room, made a complaint and demanded that we had a new midwife. Thank goodness he did, otherwise we may not have our daughter with us now.

Once organization and peace returned to the room, things calmed down. Suddenly our baby's heart beat dropped to virtually nothing (was it due to the stress of the overdose? Nobody has answered us), the room was full of people and my thoughts were: "No, not after all we've been through, NO!" Dan was pushed over to one corner of the room and we just helplessly gazed at each other, our eyes just said it all "we're going to lose our precious baby". She was a fighter though and came back to us. Shortly afterwards I was prepared for a caesarean section, but I eventually had a forceps delivery. If you look at the photos of me with our daughter straight after the birth, my mind and soul look dead. It's as though I've been in a major accident, I was numb and in shock, no smiles or tears of joy just an air of deadness. No wonder I had great problems bonding with her. The aftercare was just as dreadful, so I somewhat prematurely, discharged myself later that day with our beautiful baby.

Our daughter was extremely unsettled and hard to breast feed due to her traumatic birth. I was down from the word go and I can remember my GP visiting me and saying: "Pull yourself together, you've nothing to feel miserable about, she could have had Downs Syndrome". For starters this is an outrageously derogatory comment to make towards individuals with such special needs, whilst completely dismissing and belittling my own thoughts and feelings. I also had to go and stay in Portsmouth for two weeks during this period and we moved flats, both of which were not a great idea.

The low mood spiralled downwards into full-blown depression. I naturally swapped GPs, the second of whom was great and I had a very supportive health visitor. Nothing, however, seemed to help yet I was never admitted to hospital, because despite my feelings and lack of bonding, my baby care was deemed 'excellent'. I just didn't feel right. I knew I loved her deep down somewhere, but there was absolutely no gush of emotion. I seemed to be completely in a muddle all of the time, out of control and never organized. I was paranoid someone would take her from me, or she would die from Sudden Infant Death syndrome. Again, I was lethargic, unable to concentrate, morbid, always crying and as normal I turned to alcohol (I had given up on the breast feeding by then). Despite my GP's greatest efforts and many medication changes, it was decided that we would need a compassionate transfer to Portsmouth. It really did help being amongst my extended family even my dad was brilliant. Also, through my GP who supported alternative therapies, I saw a great homeopath. Over a few months he had me back on my feet and off my antidepressants.

We did make a formal complaint against the midwife concerned. The official reply stated that due to the midwife being out in the community for such a long time, she was out of practice with hospital policy and equipment. Also she would receive further training before returning to work. All I could think was that it was a bit bloody late to help us three. We started the motions to take legal action, with a solid case to put forward, but eventually decided it would be more painful to extend the agony of it. We wanted to leave the experience behind us and get on with our lives. It was now a case of a new home and a fresh start. I did feel as though the midwife had been 'road-tested' on us; if only she'd had the guts to be honest and admit she was out of her depth and didn't know how to use the equipment. Sometimes I think yet again, what if? So much could have been different, but then what will be will be.

Once I was over this experience I think I had another stable time in my life (relatively speaking of course) and I discovered that I was pregnant again, on the same day that Princess Diana was killed. Dan was away at sea for the last five months of my pregnancy. Again, I battled with the tentacles of depression, I just found it so difficult looking after a toddler, being heavily pregnant and with my partner away. Dan came home about 3 days before the birth of our son and boy, did I look different compared to the last time he had seen me! After an emergency caesarean, which was heaven compared to our last nightmare, our son was born weighing in at almost 10lbs. Dan was then shore-based in Portsmouth and although I was continually battling between depression and what I thought was nervous energy, I was able to keep things under control. Our next posting was Plymouth and this is where my mental health problems catapulted out of this world.

CHAPTER NINE – UNCHARTED WATERS

Following a family Christmas in Portsmouth we had to pack up our entire belongings and head west to Plymouth. I remember very little of this upheaval apart from one short space in time on the morning of our move when I was lying in bed in Drake's mess feeding my son and wondering what life had in store for us. However, these expectations were surpassed in every shape and form to the reality that lay ahead of us and I don't mean in a positive way.

I know Dan went off to sea almost immediately and although I got on with our neighbours and had enrolled my daughter in a playgroup, I was extremely lonely. I would stand looking out of the window over the valley wishing that the lights I could see were those of Portsmouth. I continued with this existence occasionally having Dan home until I knew the waves of depression were overwhelming me. Apparently, by March I was sitting in my GP's office being started on antidepressants and having a referral made for me to see the practice Community Psychiatric Nurse (CPN). I can also vaguely remember seeing the health visitor and being urged to join the local postnatal depression support group.

Towards the summer Dan was starting to get more shore-based time and we began to socialize again. I know we also spent a lot of time with my oldest sister Clare as she only lived an hour away, incidentally she proved to be a great source of help and support during the following months. I'm not sure when these sociable experiences swapped over to hypomania, all I truly know is that they definitely did and of course this knowledge is in hindsight so I was unaware of it at the time. Suddenly my life became a whirlwind of parties, alcohol and late nights or I should say early mornings! It also needs to be remembered that I was looking after two young children and the day to day running of the house.

The circle we mixed in was made up of Dan's fellow officers and some of their partners. We would meet up in bars and pubs; occasionally go out for meals but a lot of the time we went on to clubs. I would quite often carry on to the clubs with everyone else whilst Dan would go home and relieve the babysitter. Yet again I became extremely sociable, energetic, the life and soul of the party and very much aware of my sexuality. We ended up doing a barbecue for the whole wardroom and one of the junior officers called Tom had come round early to help out. We had spent a lot of time with Tom both out partying and also for meals at home, really he had become one of the family. On the evening of the barbecue we went to the supermarket together whilst Dan remained at home sorting the garden out. I just suddenly opened my eyes and realized there was a sexual chemistry between us; I had recognized these types of feelings before from my sailing days. At first I felt quite embarrassed and reserved about this non-verbal communication.

The barbecue went really well and the food went down a treat. I spent a lot of time talking with the Captain because as is often the case at these functions the senior managers can find themselves alone. Everyone left in the early hours. Dan went to bed whilst Tom and I sat talking. Of course the inevitable happened and we ended up kissing. The next day I felt confused but in some way excited, however I did receive a strange phone call from the Captain saying that we (as in myself and the Captain) would have to be careful, as people would start talking about us! So somewhat bemusedly I discussed this with Dan. Somehow I had found myself in these two charged situations.

I can't remember the exact movements of my affair with Tom, only that we had a full-blown on-going relationship, which was conducted right under Dan's nose. I can remember feeling extremely happy and excited with Tom and not at all fazed by the dangerous risks we took. If anything this fuelled my fire more intensely. I found myself living on a knife-edge and I fed off of all the anxiety it created. Suddenly I awoke sexually, believing that I was extremely attractive and had become very desirable. I guess this was just history repeating itself. I do know that for most or our encounters I was drunk, so my destructive love affair with alcohol was rearing its ugly head again.

The whole affair lasted only weeks, with Tom spending increasing amounts of time at our house. It was pretty obvious that Dan would find out and it was all over just after my thirtieth birthday at the end of August. Dan of course became suspicious and after pretending to go to bed he had listened outside the lounge one night to our conversation. Apparently, we were discussing the notion of Tom and I taking the children up to Birmingham to live. This idea seems completely incredulous to me now.

Dan demanded that Tom was to leave and he banned us both from making any contact with each other again.

I dare say Dan and I discussed the whole situation at the time but I don't recall it. We have however discussed it since and we both believe that I was in a hypomanic state, based on my behaviour before and during the affair. Dan has since had to go to sea with Tom, which must have been bloody awkward. The only part that I can truly say that attracted and stimulated me for some reason was the risk. I became addicted to it and desperately needed it, which all reduces down to a manic episode. I fed off of the roller coaster of emotions and although I thought the world of Tom it wasn't love and never would have been. I just shudder at the thought that I may have moved to Birmingham with Tom and then suddenly have come out of the mania wondering what the hell had happened. I'm glad that I didn't screw up his life as well. I'm one of the lucky ones, I often hear about individuals that have destroyed their relationships and families due to this illness.

You may be wondering why I've included such a sensitive subject in my book, especially as not many people are aware of it. I've not made this decision lightly and it has been very uncomfortable to write and will be for others to read. The reason I have decided to include this part is to highlight the degree and diversity to which Bipolar can affect an individual. Through this illness some people have lost their loved ones, families and homes. How many other illnesses can creep out and damage or overwhelm such varying sections of their mental health and life? Maybe this will give the reader thought to realize how soul destroying it can be. It's very hard to get others to accept the fact that such situations as I've described can be the direct result of Bipolar Disorder, maybe this will be able to open some people's eyes to the devastation it can cause both directly and indirectly.

I imagine that our lives would have been difficult between Dan and I whilst we rebuilt the bridges and relayed the trust between us. It was even recorded in my GP's notes that we had marital problems in the August. I think from here I entered the other half of the Bipolar equation i.e. a deep depression. By January I had fallen into a bottomless pit with my mood spiralling downwards out of control, so I was referred to a Consultant Psychiatrist for assessment. The symptoms I presented with at the consultation were as follows: depression, lethargy, tiredness, high anxiety and a variable mood. Poor sleep, poor concentration, a low self-esteem and constant thoughts of suicide. The result of this was that I was admitted there and then only being allowed to return home for some belongings. I was so scared, as although I had previously worked on psychiatric units, this time I was a patient and didn't know what the hell to expect. I was given a single room on this admission and I can remember standing there looking around in disbelief and crying as if I'd never stop. I hated being apart from my children but at the same time I knew I was really ill, the whole situation seemed unbelievable to me and I couldn't get my head around it. I can't describe these experiences in order as my memory is not only limited but also jumbled. I can remember the ward layout and a couple of the other clients, but none of the ward nursing staff or doctors apart from my consultant and very few events. I will yet again have to discuss the issues that evolved around both my inpatient stays and out patient experiences.

Right lets get the chart out and see if we can navigate some of these waters. In total I was admitted to Glenbourne psychiatric unit at Derriford hospital three times. My first admission was for a period of just under two months from 27/01/00 to 16/03/00; the second from 08/02/01 to 15/03/01 just over a month and finally from 01/05/01 to 24/05/01 just over three weeks. The first two admissions were classified as emergencies and were due to depression and severe suicidal ideation, whilst my third was more planned in nature and was due to over medicating in the community.

My suicidal ideations were mainly centred on jumping from a window, but I also had desires to take overdoses, to hang myself and to cut myself. Whilst I was in hospital I would become reclusive, isolate myself from the rest of the ward and become very quiet as though I was thinking of somehow escaping my situation. From reading my notes and listening to my heart I think the three main issues throughout all of these admissions were obsessional thoughts, agitation and my feelings of frustration and desperation.

I think we will cover the obsessional thoughts to start with. These weren't isolated to the admissions, but were quite often one of the main reasons I was admitted from home. All I wanted to do was jump out of the window or off of the stairs so that I could kill myself. Whilst I was at home I had to have twenty-four hour supervision to prevent me from achieving these goals. This meant I was constantly followed around the house even at night. As I was such a poor sleeper I would be up at least half a dozen times. So Dan, my mum, or mother-in-law depending on who was around at the time would follow me throughout the house. At one point my mother-in-law had to sleep on the floor outside my room to keep me safe. The window keys were taken away and my drugs were locked in Dan's car. I think I managed to exhaust everyone; I'm amazed and humbled by their dedication and staying power. However, I was always scheming and plotting as to when I could grab my next chance.

One of my admissions was the result of not only the depression but also the fact that I couldn't be kept safe anymore. Dan had to take a lot of time off from work to be with me and when this wasn't possible he would have to take me with him. I can remember sitting in his office, it had a big chart or map on the wall, thinking 'what has happened to me? How could I be reduced to this? I'm such a failure.'

I did actually succeed in my jumping attempts. It was a short while before we moved to Portsmouth, so in fact I was meant to be reasonably well. I'd been drinking, Dan was asleep and I just felt utterly compelled to jump. Our stairs backed up on themselves so from the banister at the top there was a clear drop to the bottom. I didn't hesitate I just climbed over the top let my legs dangle and thought, 'this is it' and jumped! I landed on the hall floor and all I had done was hurt my ankle. Ok I thought, let's try again, hopefully it will be second time lucky! I repeated it all over again, without the desired results, instead I just had even more pain in my ankles, which cut straight through the alcohol. The next day I could hardly walk, not surprisingly I didn't want to go to Casualty, so Dan took me to a small medical centre. I didn't let them know any of my psychiatric history or current medications and I refused to let them know how I did it as there was no way I wanted to go back into hospital.

I did get a lot of help with regards to these obsessional thoughts mainly from a doctor who was doing Cognitive Analytical Therapy (CAT) with me and from my Community Psychiatric Nurse. I actively used the following methods to try and break the chain: relaxation tapes, distraction, getting out of the house, spending time with the children, sleeping, working through handouts, hitting a newspaper on the floor, writing down negative thoughts and setting small achievable goals. So you can see that despite the severity of my illness I still worked very hard to regain some control; this the reader will discover later in the book is something that was not feasible during my hospital stays in Portsmouth due to the extreme levels of my medication. I have found that throughout my life no matter how severe the circumstances are a part of me will keep on trying to fight, to survive; as long as my senses and mind are not numbed by too much medication. As an alternative to hospital admission, attempts were made for me to attend a day hospital but unfortunately there were not enough spaces.

However as I've just mentioned I saw a fantastic doctor who did CAT with me at least once a week. She was an amazing women, having experienced so much in life and was able to teach, show and share with me so many things about myself and my past (albeit often very painful) that has been invaluable even to this day. I also had an awful lot of support from Kate my CPN, both in hospital and at home; I think she is definitely the best CPN I have ever come across. On top of this I would attend a clinic when home to do things such as aromatherapy, it may sound good but I hated it. Everyone seemed really ill and inappropriate and I just thought, shit is this what my life will be like from now on? In hospital I had a few sessions at the day hospital, a lot of occupational therapy input and there was talk of me doing Cognitive Behavioural Therapy to ease/resolve my obsessive thoughts. Although I'm not sure if the latter happened! At times it would seem that my thoughts were viewed as having a psychotic element. This is because I would describe periodically having a man's voice outside of my head telling me to jump. Fortunately, I don't remember this.

The next big issue is that I experienced severe agitation both in and out of hospital. I would try really hard in hospital with relaxation and distraction but I could not get a release from it. My body would shake, my heart race and my breath quicken. This wouldn't just be a short panic attack but would actually last for hours and although I desperately wanted to I couldn't escape it. I frequently requested and received 'as required medication' to alleviate it. I don't think all of the staff members were happy to dispense it, which would make me really angry as I was prescribed it legitimately and I always tried alternative methods of alleviation first. When at home during one of these periods my depression seemed to be lifting but my agitation got worse by the day. I ended up on a drug called Clopixol and would increase the dosage myself to try and gain some relief. However, I did suffer with bad side effects and managed to wean myself off it as I have frequently achieved in my life with numerous other drugs. I do laugh now though as my last Plymouth admission was mainly due to the large levels of Benzodiazepines that I was on. On admission I was taking 25mg of Diazepam (a tranquilliser) and Temazepams (sleeping tablets). These were viewed as excessive yet shortly after my discharge from St James' (Portsmouth) I was on 90mg of Diazepam; a big difference don't you think?

I became increasingly frustrated, as my depression seemed difficult to treat and was very slow at responding. I had numerous drug changes and couldn't understand why they weren't working. My feelings would turn inwards and I would often wonder why I had to suffer like this and for such a long time. It would leave me with a whole bag of emotions not only of guilt at being ill and a poor mother, but also wanting to just end it all. I guess again I longed for peace of mind, body and soul. I would often state that all I wanted was to get better quickly, but failing that the only other option I could see was death. I often ended up drowning in a river of tears. I think the frustration and desperation is what led me to agreeing to Electro Convulsive Therapy (ECT) as I just wanted to get better quickly and this seemed like a last ditched attempt. I had seen ECT performed when I was a student nurse; the patient had a bad reaction, which left my mind full of horrific and degrading images. So for me to actually agree to ECT was huge. Before each session (I had eight in total) I had visions of what I would look like, which turned my stomach and numbed my soul. I also got very frustrated with this treatment, as although my mood would be elevated it was very short lived. Each time a glimpse of happiness was on the horizon, there would be a crash down which became intolerable. I also experienced short-term memory problems, which although this was an incomparable side affect in relation to the depression it remained difficult to deal with. In my notes it states that I needed ECT as 'an emergency life saving procedure and due to failed drug treatment.' So I guess from a medical viewpoint there was a reason to have it. At some point along the line I also had the mood stabilizer Lithium added to the cocktail of medication that I was on. This was meant to augment the antidepressants.

As I was suicidal I was started off on observations of fifteen minutes, which would then extend to thirty minutes until eventually the staff only needed to know where I was at all times. These seem like very set procedures as my mood would fluctuate, deteriorating greatly in the evenings. I was allowed out on home leave but it was on the understanding that I was with someone who could take responsibility for me all times. However, as I already mentioned I was constantly plotting and scheming and I managed to take overdoses on two different occasions.

The first attempt, according to my notes, was after I had gone out to lunch with Dan. We went home and I searched for the tablets without Dan knowing. When I got back to the ward I told the staff and had to go to Casualty by ambulance. They managed to get hold of Dan and he spent the remainder of the evening with me.

Referring back to my notes, the reason I had notified the staff was purely because I hadn't said good-bye to my children. The second attempt occurred whilst I was on overnight leave. I'd been drinking and had taken an overdose of four different types of drugs at midnight. I had gone to bed and slept until ten the next morning at which point I vomited and was incontinent of urine. Following this I experienced visual hallucinations (one of which involved hundreds of hedgehogs in the back garden) and continued to shake until 8p.m. of that evening. Yet again I hadn't told Dan and the only reason I did tell the staff was because my CAT therapist said I should. I described my feelings then as those of being a failure and being tired of continually fighting. So I guess it was another scenario of playing Russian roulette with my life, as having gone to bed I hadn't expected to wake up.

With all of this going on the security of Dan's job was waning, he had taken so much time off from work despite having a lot of naval support. We had been allocated a naval social worker and had subsequently received help from a naval support worker. She would help out with the children, take them to school and the naval nursery and collect them at the end of the day. However the children were becoming increasingly upset, especially my son. When I went into hospital for the first time, I had to abruptly stop breast-feeding my son due to the fact that we were apart and I had been put on medication. He became quite distant from me whilst my daughter was unsettled along with the emotions of my illness I found both of them difficult to deal with. I guess the whole situation was just too much for them to cope with. On top of this Dan had been informed that if he were to get called back from sea again he would lose his job. On the basis of this information the decision was made to take a compassionate move back to Portsmouth.

Another issue that needs to be mentioned here are my hormonal problems. My doctor in Plymouth first suspected it and a referral was made for me on the basis that when I didn't have periods my mood was greatly improved. I was started on a course of Zoladex injections, which stops the menstrual cycle occurring and Hormone Replacement Therapy. Although this combination was stopped for a time in the Portsmouth hospital I have remained on this regime up to the present day and even though I am now considering a more permanent approach this treatment has definitely helped me and made a difference to my life. I also officially had my diagnosis label changed whilst here. On my first admission I was classified as having 'Post-Natal Depression' but by my second I was classified as having 'Severe Resistant Depression.' Well that label list is definitely growing by the chapter!

I also had a lot of worries during this period which I feel should be taken into consideration, although apparently I reacted 'normally' to them! As already mentioned there was the impending move to Portsmouth, however we did also move house whilst in Plymouth which didn't help. The fear of Dan losing his job was great. If that had happened we would have been without a home or financial security. Also my aunty died following a long battle with renal cancer at a young age. I had always been very close to her as she and my uncle had lived across the road from my parents. I loved her dearly and she had always been a great source of advice and comfort throughout my troubled teenage years as well as the subsequent ones. I don't think I really grieved for her until I was well enough, which was long after my Portsmouth hospital discharge. Up until then I had always been too ill or drugged to get in touch with my emotions. I have never stopped missing her and I don't think I ever will. Finally, Sue experienced a nasty accident and severely fractured her arm. She needed surgery, a hospital stay and much physiotherapy, yet as always she kept us all going.

The last area I want to cover is that of mania. This word wasn't used at all in my Portsmouth notes neither as an in-patient or an outpatient, however I have found it here in my Plymouth records. The first extract is from a letter written by my consultant to my GP, in December 2000: 'She tells me that her depression has improved dramatically over the past two weeks, but the problem for her now is one of agitation. It sounds as though she might be going slightly manic because she describes rushing around every day, a feeling that she's racing, feeling happy and marked episodes of shaking. She is not sleeping well at present because of all this, but I note she is not eating to excess or spending excess money.' Following this appointment my mood stabilizers (I was on two) were increased and my antidepressant decreased in an attempt to control the mania.

This second extract is again taken from a letter written by my consultant to my GP, in January 2001: 'my impression is that she is stable at present. The depression has lifted and there is no evidence of mania.' Now I completely understand and appreciate that Bipolar is a very difficult illness to diagnose, but when there was such an apparent episode why wasn't it questioned further? Maybe someone should have sat back and observed the whole picture including the past, rather then just seeing the depression and no further. If I had been diagnosed correctly back then I wouldn't have had to grasp at the surface gasping for air, whilst the turbulent waves crashed over me. I know mania was never an option whilst I was in Portsmouth, until now that is.

Finally, I am on the correct medication which I have responded well to, consequently I am healthy and leading a normal life. Maybe health professionals need to keep their eyes open and not just focus on the previous 'correct' diagnosis, but instead look beyond that point and over the horizon. Yet again I guess it is a case of what if, but as I'm too fully aware now what will be will be. So on to Portsmouth and the invading foggy seas.

CHAPTER TEN – FOGGY SEAS

Yet again I find myself desperate to put pencil to paper and process my thoughts into words. However, this time my thoughts are extremely jumbled, infused with pain and full of confusion. This chapter will take the reader through a stormy passage of my in patient stays in St James Psychiatric Hospital, Portsmouth. I cannot write these experiences in chronological order, as my memories of this time are so poor due to the illness, medication and ECT. I would have to rely solely on my notes, which would result in a factual account void of all emotions. I do remember some of my feelings and thoughts though and as I read through my clinical notes people and events start to become a little clearer. At this stage I have no idea how I will write this chapter or the style that I will choose. I think all I can do is let my thoughts flow freely on certain issues and hope the outcome is of some value.

I know that I wanted to sit and cry when I shared my Bath experiences with you. However, the key word there was wanted, this time half way through reading my notes all my resolves dissolved into water. I had no control and the silent tears poured endlessly down my face, like the sea flowing from around the world's oceans. I would not allow myself to sob, I didn't want to give in to the bitter memories but I had no control over the silent tears as they just kept on coming, driven by an unseen force. I think I cried for the lost year of my life, for the pitiful creature I had become back then and for all the pain and distress I had experienced. Before I read my notes I felt very aggrieved by all the nursing and medical staff, believing my situation was entirely their fault. However I now know that wasn't entirely the case, well not on a personal level; although I do believe one could challenge the establishment and resources.

When we moved to Portsmouth I managed to remain at home for ten days, before I needed an urgent assessment and was consequently admitted to hospital on the 10/07/01. This admission lasted until the 18/09/01, a total of just over two months. I was then readmitted again after only nine days and this time I remained in hospital until the 19/08/02 which meant I was an in patient for just under eleven months and thus a grand total of thirteen months. This is a huge part of a person's life to lose, especially as a large proportion of it I cannot remember. That feeling is extremely scary, how do you deal with such a big memory and life loss?

It wasn't until I read these notes that I discovered two really important pieces of information. I am aware that both of these events occurred but I had no idea when or what it was like. Firstly as I've already mentioned, my auntie who I was extremely close to died of renal cancer whilst I was in Plymouth. Until now, although I can remember the phone call and the funeral I had no idea when it had happened. Secondly, Mum was diagnosed with having breast cancer, which meant she underwent both surgery and radiotherapy. It seems that when she was first diagnosed I was aware of her condition, but beyond that point I had no recognition or understanding of the fact. I don't remember any of her treatment, illness or distressing recovery. This causes me so much hurt that although not alone, my mum went through all of this with no acknowledgement from me let alone any love, help or support. How can I ever make that up to her? Incidentally, my parents also had a new house built and moved into it during this period and I have absolutely zero memories of these events.

Right life jackets and harnesses on we need to enter this foggy sea. As written in my notes my diagnosis was 'Recurrent Resistant Depressive Illness' (yet another label) and my condition was frequently referred to as being severe. I'll try to summarize generally what my symptoms were on my admissions. I was very low in mood, had very poor motivation, concentration and eye contact. My sleep was disturbed, my appetite was poor, I experienced high levels of anxiety and was very tearful. Apparently, I also looked flat, expressionless and miserable with low self-esteem. Again one of my main problems was my self-harm and suicidal thoughts with active intentions. The methods I was preoccupied with at that time were jumping out of windows/cars, overdoses and wanting to cut my wrists with a knife.

I can remember my first night of admission as I was followed around constantly (obviously on a one to one with the nurse). I found this extremely intrusive and I remember sitting on the toilet with a nurse outside the door not understanding why she was there, but in the same breathe I was searching every possible route to killing myself; so I guess that answers that question. From this ward I went onto the intensive care unit (ICU) where I had a nurse constantly with me. Apparently I was very withdrawn, isolated myself from staff and clients, and remained in my bed space for long periods of time. I hated this place and I do remember that we even had to ask for teaspoons when making a drink as they were classified as 'potentially dangerous weapons'! I remember the atmosphere on the ward was constantly charged as though everyone was waiting for the next client to 'kick off'. I also have this vague recollection that a male client smashed a window and I can remember feeling very frightened. I know I had several visitors but the only ones that come to mind are my cousins and uncle. They definitely did not like it on the ward and had also picked up on the electric atmosphere. I also find it very strange that although I can remember the complete layout of the ward, I don't remember any of the other clients or staff, none of their names or faces.

I stayed on the first ward for two nights and I have included extracts from my notes, which highlight examples of the suicidal thoughts that I was having: 'Lorraine has continued on 1:1 nursing obs. She has remained quiet and appears preoccupied. Lorraine has just approached me to say she has an overwhelming desire to hang herself in the bathroom with her dressing gown belt. Distraction methods used... Careful observations required at all times.' 'Lorraine has continued on 1:1 nursing obs... Lorraine approached and said she felt she wanted to jump over the banister of the stairs and said the only thing that stopped her was knowing I was standing next to her. Given 1: 1 time... Transferred to ICU.' It does seem that my most dangerous and intense suicide thoughts occurred when I could switch off all feelings towards my children, as when this happened there was nothing to stop me from committing the act.

Whilst I was on the Intensive Care Unit and according to my notes previously, I experienced voices telling me to hurt myself. I also tried to take the mirror off the bathroom wall in an attempt to cause some damage to myself. I fail to remember either of these occurrences. I stayed on this ward for ten days and was then moved to Ellen Cook ward, my heaven or more appropriately prison, where I spent the majority of the next thirteen months of my life. This transfer from wards was due to 'bed pressure', rather then assessment or concern for my medical state. Was it the appropriate move? Now I have to match the fragments of my memory to the information I have read in my notes and hopefully I will be able to piece together my experiences.

One of my biggest issues here was an obsession with jumping out of the window. I would repeatedly spend time trying to force the windows, break the safety restraints, destroy the locks and remove the chains. I know I desperately wanted to die and frantically with my vision I tried to find a way to achieve this. The only options I came up with were the windows. To start with, the staff were not aware and I would go from toilet to bathroom to bedroom trying to succeed in my mission. I would then try and do the 'right' thing and confide in the staff my intensions, usually after I had been balancing on one of the window ledges. I spent the large proportion of my stay here under observations of fifteen minutes due to my suicidal intensions and desires to abscond, then only occasionally and not until nearer the end of my stay were these increased to thirty-minute observations and then eventually no regimented observations at all. Although I was allowed on home leave, I was not to be left alone and when I returned to the ward I would go back onto observations of fifteen minutes. Quite often my home leave was cancelled due to my state of mind and the intensions I had for when I left the ward. This is an extract from my notes illustrating my obsession with jumping: 'On leaving the ward the HCSW observed Lorraine at bathroom window, returned to ward and alerted staff. Bathroom was entered; Lorraine was sat up on the window ledge trying to climb out. Tearful and distressed, did not want to get down stated she wanted to jump. Assisted down… fed up with feeling this way – just wants peace… and observed each time she went to the toilet. Continued to express her determination to succeed in jumping out of the window and stated she would pick a time when staff were distracted.'

Following this my bed was moved to a safer place, I was observed when entering the bathrooms and received support and one to one time with the nursing staff. However I still continued to hear the 'voices' telling me to jump, so I made several attempts and became obsessed with succeeding. I also got extremely suicidal in the evenings. Even my daughter made me a lavender bag to put under my pillow to 'stop me jumping'. This is another revelation and it breaks my heart. How did she know? What did she think?

With all these issues during the acute stage of my illness my memory is very strange. I have a vague recollection of the above, but when I try to remember more it's as though I am looking down a very long, dark tunnel with just a glimpse of light at the end. When I focus on this light I get a glimmer of the memory, as though it feels familiar but I can't quite see no matter how bold my efforts are. I know people that have near death experiences talk of this analogy, maybe it is similar but I know that is exactly how it feels for me and is the only way I can attach words or meaning to it.

Another big concern during these admissions was my sleep patterns. It's a bit of the chicken and the egg scenario! I experienced very poor sleep at night and found it difficult to get off to sleep; I would suffer nightmares, was up frequently throughout the night and would wake early in the mornings. However at some point in the equation I would go back to bed and would stay asleep for the majority of the day. It appears that the staff tried hard to keep me awake during the day, with continual explanations that if I slept all day I would not sleep at night. It must have been extremely frustrating for them, as I frequently ignored their prompts and advise, instead I would return to bed and remain there. I do actually remember feeling irritated that I was being constantly nagged and I could not understand their insistence. However I can also remember my own reasoning, which is upsetting and completely reflects my state of mind. I know these feelings as if they were happening now, I stayed in bed for two reasons: firstly because 'it was the closest I could get to death' and secondly because it was 'the only way I could forget it all'. These reasons are documented in my notes but I don't think anyone paid attention to them, as they were never discussed. Perhaps only I find these two statements so upsetting. I understand them as wanting a non-existence, no longer able to deal with the distress and pain, instead being desperate to enter a void. As I was unable to kill myself I retreated to the next best escapes: sleep and drugs.

I also used to keep myself isolated from both the staff and other clients, spending the majority of the time in my bed space, and visiting only the smoking rooms at times. I know this is mostly due to the depression but I also think it was because I could not quite believe that I was in a psychiatric institution yet again. If I ignored it then maybe it would all go away. Gradually as the time went past and I eventually started to improve I would mix more with the other clients and converse with the staff. However I would end up spending all my time in the smoking room, where I would get through sixty cigarettes a day and copious amounts of cola.

My motivation was so low due to the depression that all my personal hygiene needs went out of the window (a place where I longed to be!). This was because it required too much energy to perform: I had no care for appearance or aromas and to be honest I don't think I ever thought that part of my being needed attention. I would go for a few weeks without a bath or a shower and it would only occur through the guidance and encouragement of staff and then followed up with much praise from them. A prime example for my lack of concern is that I ended up in casualty having my earring studs cut out as they'd become infected and imbedded. I hadn't even thought to take them out and the same pair had been in my ears for six months. Around this time I also had to go to casualty to have my ring cut off due to my finger swelling. I gained four stone in weight during these two admissions mostly through the drugs I was on but also lack of movement and indulgence of hospital puddings rather then a balanced diet. For someone who had struggled with an eating disorder this was extremely distressing and just fuelled my depression even further. I would look in the mirror and the face of Lorry was no longer reflected.

One of my major concerns during this time and for many months after my discharge was the level of my sedation. I have always, along with my family, felt angry towards the medical team for sedating me beyond all reason. I do still believe that they should have taken a far more active role in regulating it and that I shouldn't have been reduced to the inert object that I was. I do now believe that I also played a part. I can remember the extreme levels of anxiety, to the extent that I would be violently shaking, not knowing what to do with my body or how to grasp any level of peace within my mind and soul. This is still something I treasure now, that is to have peace of mind, body and soul whilst being able to smile spontaneously. Especially in the early days, I learnt and exercised different methods of control and relaxation; these were soon replaced by the burning desire for drugs as I soon became addicted both physically and psychologically. At every opportunity I would ask for 'PRN' medication (pro re nata, a Latin term used in medical shorthand for 'as required drugs'). When staff refused or offered alternative anxiety relief I would become cross and confused, questioning them and not appreciating their rationale. I was eventually prescribed various sedating drugs due to the extreme levels of anxiety, which reached the point to where I was severely over medicated. Basically I became an empty shell just rotting away on the inside. One of the results of this action was that I ended up constantly falling over when walking, tumbling out of my bed and sliding off chairs. Which left me with very painful knocks and bruises. It reached the stage that my bed had to be moved against the wall and a mattress placed on the floor, also there was a discussion as to whether cot sides should be put on my bed. Goodness knows how many accident forms needed completing as a consequence of my falls.

Due to the sedation I was frequently incontinent of urine and faeces nocturnally, however according to my notes I never seemed disturbed by the fact, this illustrates just how detached I was from my environment. If that was to happen now I would be mortified. I also remember the confusion at night when on leaving my bed space I would not be able to find my way back and would wander aimlessly around other patients' beds, this in fact was quite frightening. Along with this I can remember reaching the toilets, sitting down, falling asleep and then wake up on the floor not knowing where I was.

Consequently I developed hip pain, was not able to walk properly and advised to use the walk in shower on another ward, as I was no longer able to bath on Ellen Cook or at home. So not only was my mental health severely suffering but also my physical well-being. My dad describes me as a 'zombie' at this time with vacant eyes and saliva dribbling from my mouth. One of the most painful truths is an event that frequently happened which my eight year old daughter has told me about on numerous occasions, asking me why? Apparently her and my son would come in to visit me, but I wouldn't recognize them. She would say "Mummy it's me *****", but all I would do is return a blank, meaningless stare void of all comprehension. How do I deal with this information? How could a mother not even recognize her own child? What must this have meant to my daughter? As a parent you always want to be there for your child, to nurture them, protect them and ultimately to love them. It is so apparent to me now that I was not able to provide any of those unconditional parental roles. This makes me feel that I let them both down, especially my little girl, as she was old enough to understand. It is something I have to live with every day and although it can be rationalized that does not take away the fact that I wasn't there for them. Even on a basic level. The only way I can live with this knowledge is to promise myself that I will never let this happen to them again. I will keep fighting for them, whilst learning as much as I can about this condition, loving them and cherishing our times together. They are my precious sunrise.

During this period of heavy sedation I also became very unwell with a resilient chest infection and the issue of premenstrual syndrome was readdressed. As my depression was proving extremely resistant despite numerous antidepressants, anti-anxiety drugs, steroidal medications and well over a dozen ECT's I was referred for a CT scan, a hormonal opinion and to see an Endocrinologist. I also ended up having an investigation to see if I had a deep vein thrombosis due to hip and knee pain. All of these investigations bar the hormonal assessment, proved to be negative, but I was to continue with Zoladex injections and HRT (to control the PMS).

During this time I was also having memory problems from the countless ECT's, at times experiencing confusion and hallucinating. I have copied this following extract from my notes: 'Lorraine has been quiet this am... After lunch approached myself to ask for clean bedding, shortly after came to the office complaining that there were lots of 'wriggly things' all over her bed. However when I got there the bed was fine. I looked under and around the bed with Lorraine and although there was clearly nothing there, Lorraine protested that she could still see them and they were wandering across the sheets'.

When I reached this point in my notes I had been reading for about two hours. As I crossed the parts where my physical health was deteriorating, experiencing confusion and memory problems my eyes welled up with tears and I had to fight myself mentally not to cry. However when I came across this passage the tears splashed on to my cheeks drop by drop, until an immense ocean ebbed from my eyes. I had no control at all, yet I made no sound just letting these silent tears cascade down my face. My thoughts were: how pitiful I was, why had such dreadful events happened in my life? What had I been reduced to? Surely this was only a scene out of an old black and white film about psychiatric institutions? However as we are all very much aware this was a modern day reality, no movie just true life as I had experienced it. It was as though hands reached out of those pages and pulled me in, so once again I was there experiencing this living hell. I felt panicky, could feel my breathing become fast and shallow, my heart rate rising and my head spinning. It took me a few hours to lift the foreboding thoughts and feelings, to control the tears and steady my breathing. I used all of the cognitive behavioural skills I had learnt to separate then from now. Although I was able to experience and appreciate those horrors I was eventually able to return them to that time, to that chapter in my life and ultimately to this chapter in my book. After all it is now only a chapter of my past and not my future.

Mum at some point during this period insisted on speaking to the ward manager and was invited to attend a ward round. She challenged my consultant that I was a fighter at heart, but all the time I was so heavily sedated none of these traits could be raised to the surface. She demanded to know how they expected me to fight for myself when I couldn't even recognize my loved ones. I can also remember sitting there, head in hands, informing my consultant that if he didn't do something soon then I definitely would. I have also since learnt that Sue took in a photograph of me grinning at a yacht's wheel during one of my sailing journeys, stating that this was the true Lorry and she wanted me back. When I read my notes it would appear there were problems with my family; me claiming they wanted the impossible i.e. for me to pull myself together and they admitting they didn't understand. However one thing I do know is that they never once stopped fighting for me or showing me unconditional love and support. For this I am eternally grateful. Following their interventions my sedatives were gradually reduced and I simultaneously started to make improvements albeit small but at least in the right direction at last.

My relationship with Dan was also deteriorating, from what I've read he was becoming irritable and cross with me, not feeling he could cope with me at home when I was so suicidal and physically unwell. It didn't help when the Au Pair started work, as I felt even more pushed out from the family and redundant in my role as a mother and wife. It appears that we argued a lot and that Dan would ignore me when I was out on home leave. The final crunch for him was my overdose. I had gone on home leave for the weekend and on the Friday night I went out with Mum and Sue for a meal and then on to the theatre. I can remember sitting in the restaurant and feeling utterly miserable deciding then that I would take my tablets but I never let anyone know my thoughts. When I returned Sue dropped me off and the house was in darkness, everyone was in bed, great I thought. Dan had been drinking (he was now relying heavily on alcohol as a stress reliever) and I finished off the remainder of his wine. I now had the courage to go through with it and I just took my remaining tablets without really thinking too much. Yet again I went to bed presuming that I would fail to wake up to another sunrise.

Dan discovered what I had done when he awoke in the morning, also finding faeces on the landing floor (I don't remember this) and rang the ward to inform them he was bringing me back. When I returned to Ellen Cook and told them what I had taken they called an ambulance and I was moved to Casualty. I stayed in hospital for two days, on an intravenous infusion and a heart monitor, as I had taken a reasonable amount of lithium. One of the nurses at Ellen Cook informed Dan that I couldn't have been serious; as I hadn't taken my Amitriptyline so that meant I was just trying to manipulate him. These words stuck with him and he has since told me that this was the reason for his refusal to see me. In actual fact I didn't realize at that time how dangerous this drug was otherwise I would have taken the whole lot, as it was I had consumed a large amount of Lithium. I know I was serious when I took the overdose, I also acknowledge the fact that it was easier to do due to the alcohol. I guess I was yet again playing Russian roulette with my life and I didn't care what the outcome would be.

The only time Dan came to see me when I was in the Medical Assessment Unit was to pick me up and take me to St James' and from this point on he refused to visit. The following extract is from my medical notes: 'Wanting to see her husband and her children but now knows her husband does not want to see her anymore and does not wish for her to return home'. I can distinctly remember lying across the chairs with my head on Mum's lap crying uncontrollably and regretting what I had done. This seemed to be a turning point for me, as I knew I desperately wanted to keep custody of my children and that I didn't want to lose them. Little by little I improved and as the sedation was decreased my fighting spirit returned. I knew I had to get strong if I didn't want to screw things up again. Dan took the children abroad for a two week holiday and although I missed them desperately this enabled us both to have time and space to think about our futures, together or apart.

Somehow over the weeks we managed to piece things together enough for me to be discharged back to our marital home. From this point it took months of turmoil, hurt and pain to be resolved before we could describe ourselves as being in an equal relationship and happily married again. My love for my children is one of the main drives that I've had to keep me going throughout the darkest and most desolate of times. When I've been so close to killing myself their two faces have appeared in my mind's eye almost taunting me saying "How could you leave us? What will our lives be like without you? How could we ever get over your death?" Then something takes over I'm not sure if it's maternal instincts, guilt or soul absorbing love. Whatever it is, this X factor has kept me alive and strong enough to get through the darkest days and stormiest nights. The times I have attempted to take my life since having them is when I've switched off from them, in that I lose their precious faces in the heavy fog of my mind. My life may be at times a raging hurricane, but their spirits are the equivalent of a calming tranquil sea. They have quite literally kept me alive.

I need to mention three different people now. The first, an amazing ward sister who mainly did nights. She was always supportive and had time to listen, two skills that couldn't be presumed of other staff. Through her kindness I was able to admit my alcohol problem honestly and openly. Consequently I was commenced on a detoxification program, which really helped with my physical withdrawal symptoms and helped me to abstain on the whole. Secondly my first Community Psychiatric Nurse called Jo. Although I do not particularly remember our meetings, through reading my notes I realize that she helped me greatly. However when I met Jo I knew I recognized her; she was a fellow student from my psychology degree course. I feel so unsettled about this now. I remember being aware of her face, but not having the cognitive prowess to tell someone who she was and that I was uncomfortable about it. She was younger then me (I had been classified as a mature student whilst studying my degree) and although I knew her from the past she hadn't been a friend. Now she knows intimate details about my past and present and has seen me at my worst. All I can say is it makes me feel embarrassed and small. Finally, I don't remember my occupational therapist at all but it would appear she did extremely valuable work with me. We covered areas such as anxiety management and alternative ways of coping to medication; motivation involving methods in caring for personal hygiene accompanied by great support and praise when completed; concentration skills such as reading, conversations and television; exercise and mobility skills in that she helped me find safe methods of moving around and sleeping and living with my pronounced shaking and encouraging small amounts of exercise to help with my weight loss.

At the beginning of this chapter I have written how my family and myself felt let down by St James Hospital. I strongly believe that I was completely over medicated, but there were no alternative therapies established to help with this scenario. In my recent admission to the private hospital I was taught how to deal with self-harm, suicide, anxiety and depression through cognitive therapy. In the private hospital I would see the psychologist twice weekly and each day I would attend support groups guided by therapists and covering a wide range of subjects. Hence I wasn't sedated and I learnt many invaluable skills, which I use on a daily basis now. I was discharged within five weeks of my admission, which says a lot to me. The only type of therapy that I received whilst at St James' was through my one or two weekly visits by the occupational therapist. Surely when people are challenged by their mental health, then psychological therapies should be available on a frequent and regular basis to all. Treatment should not be left solely to medication, Electro Convulsive Therapy and in my case it would seem to chance alone.

The thought that sends a knife through my heart is that there could be someone else just like I was, sitting in that ward suffering in the same undignified way. This creates such anguish for me and I desperately want to help in some way, so hopefully this book could fulfil part of that wish. If it does then all the distress and pain I have been through would adopt some meaning and to a greater degree would have been worth it. I need to restate the title of this book 'there will always be a sunrise', the semantics behind this being that no matter what is happening today there will always be a new sunrise tomorrow and the start of a new day brings new hope. Although today maybe shit, who knows what tomorrow may bring. This is how I endeavour to experience life and it certainly makes a difference to me and enables me to fulfil my desire of inner peace and happiness. I hope this helps!

CHAPTER ELEVEN – THE STARS ABOVE AND THE SEA BELOW

Right now we're at the point in this passage where I was officially discharged from St James hospital. This by no way means that I was cured or healthy, in fact the truth is far from that. In some ways the next seven months were even harder then the year I had spent in hospital. Each time I write a chapter I tend to brainstorm, which results in a sheet of A4 on the table in front of me covered in titles. This time I seem to have run out of space and I don't know where to start in fear that it will become disjointed.

I was discharged in the August of 2002 and I don't think I showed any signs of improvement until about February 2003 at which time I just headed back towards health at a steady pace. One of my main problems during this period was my Diazepam abuse and my intake reached ludicrously high levels. At one point I was on 60mgs of Diazepam with an extra 60mgs when I required it (PRN). At another time it states in my notes that I was on 45mgs of Diazepam plus a PRN dose, which in fact was the result of halving my intake. A further section describes that I had an accumulative intake of 70mgs throughout one day and I had become anxious, as I couldn't work out which room was which in my house so I took a further amount of Diazepam. A final example is when I telephoned the out of hours Assessment and Support Team (AST). On this occasion I had taken 20mgs of Diazepam during the day and then polished off another 50mgs in a single dose that evening, but this was not a suicide attempt. The reason I've written these figures is to highlight the vast amount that I was taking on a regular basis.

This obviously affected me both physically and mentally. I will now copy from my notes a section that was written by my CPN to highlight this issue: 'She presents almost incoherent and admits to abusing her Diazepam, stating she has already taken 40mgs this morning and will take more this afternoon. I advised her about the adverse effects of all her medication and the amount she is taking and explained that this is why she presents so shaky and unable to talk coherently, with very poor memory. Lorraine is also wetting the bed on occasions and has fallen several times at home.' I expect you're wondering why I was taking so much. I think originally it started as a means to manage the agitation, from that point onwards I discovered that I was able to use the drug to become detached from not only the environment I was in but also myself and at that time I found both of these components intolerable. After that and especially on these extreme levels I became both physically and psychologically addicted.

I would have to walk with a stick as I was constantly falling over. At one point I fell down the stairs at home and had to go to Casualty via an ambulance. At night I would often wander around the house into the others' rooms and I even managed to get hold of a bottle of bleach but luckily as I was so drugged despite my best efforts I was unable to get the lid off. I would have drunk it in my sedated stupor. As stated my memory was poor, my words mumbled and I had very little awareness as to what was going on around me. I was threatened with another hospital admission purely to reduce my Diazepam intake. Somehow in very small amounts and extremely slowly at first I was able to start reducing the amounts, whilst remaining in the community. I was only allowed this prescription from my psychiatrist and on a weekly basis so in that way he was able to keep a very close eye on the situation. It wasn't easy, as I had to deal with quite bad withdrawal effects including shaking and agitation. I used to go to a gym on a regular basis and can remember the restaurant staff having to carry my drink to the table as I shook too much to hold it and they provided me with a straw so I was able to take a sip. It was ironic really that I had originally taken the drug for agitation and once I started coming off it that is exactly what I suffered with, so basically I gained nothing but lost a lot i.e. my existence.

During this time I also had explorations into back pain supposedly from all the falls, but this turned out to have a 'significant non-organic component' and that I was tending to 'somatacise' the symptoms. So I guess my psyche had a lot to answer for. I don't really remember the early days of my Diazepam reduction, I know from my notes that I got stuck on 45mgs for quite a while. However after that I can remember feeling quite determined that I would succeed and I even kept a chart on the fridge to monitor my progress. I think as per normal whilst the drug induced fog lifted from my brain my fighting spirit came back with a vengeance. It was a slow process just dropping by 5mgs a week, but I finally reached my goal in March 2003 and this is very coincidental as it was around this time that I actually started to take positive steps towards my recovery. From then onwards I was desperate to reduce the remainder of my medication, which I succeeded in doing with one of my antidepressants; but was told I had to continue with the remaining antidepressant and the lithium.

Right what's next, the bad apple I think, my suicidal thoughts. In the first few months following my discharge I continued to be extremely suicidal, it basically remained an ongoing battle and at times I was nearly readmitted because of it. I wasn't obsessed with jumping during those months but instead overdoses, cutting my wrists and stabbing myself in the liver. I think the latter was because I knew I would be able to bleed to death quite quickly. This is a quote from my notes, which portrays the suicidal ideation: 'She described making plans last week to go to Portsdown hill with a bottle of wine, all of her tablets and to slit her wrists.' During these times I used the AST team an awful lot yet I would often be very quite and reluctant to talk once I'd phoned them. They would state in their reports that it would be difficult to hear my voice, to engage with me and that I would communicate in a depressed tone. Yet again my love for my children prevented me from taking my life as was stated by the CPN: 'The only thing that stops her ending her life, is to look at her children when they are asleep.' This is repeated over and over again throughout my notes, however I did find a very disturbing piece of information. I find this extremely difficult to write about as in a way this means I am admitting to having had these thoughts which is shocking: '…. admitting to wanting to stab herself in the liver. Lorraine then admitted to wanting to stab her children as she felt this would be better for them not to suffer her death. Lorraine admitted to having these thoughts in the past and describes them as fleeting thoughts. Lorraine is aware that Social Services may have to get involved if these thoughts become more frequent and I advised her of the management of this risk.' So what can I now say apart from I'm lost for words. Did I really consider taking my children's priceless lives from them? I guess I can see a little of the thinking in that I didn't want them to suffer any pain as a result of my death. To be honest though I do wonder if there is an element of selfishness in that I couldn't face leaving them behind. This passage is a constant revelation to me, and is full of many disturbing disclosures.

Putting these discoveries aside, it appears that as my condition started to improve I greatly enjoyed being with the children and caring for them. I was concerned about my son at one point as he was hitting himself and had some minor problems at school. I engaged the help of a Paediatric nurse from my surgery and together we helped him express his feelings and worries over a few weeks. Now apart from a few, minor, boyish antics he has developed in to a well-adjusted loving child. It also materializes that there were problems with my family, as I seemed to feel they didn't understand my illness or me and continually wanted me to 'pull myself together'. I find this difficult to believe, but maybe through my drugged mind that was how I perceived the situation. I know both my CPN and Consultant provided a lot of input especially by including them in team meetings. I know they always listened to my family's concerns and tried to provide support, however I also know the promised care often fell short which was frustrating for both my family and myself. It would appear from my notes that my CPN was very professional and helpful, but we all remember her letting me down whilst her demeanor was that of a very flustered individual who was unable to cope. I also felt at times I had a greater knowledge then she did.

So that's nearly all of the relationships covered except for a very important one and that was between Dan and myself. I don't know where to start here as it wasn't good and to a certain extent I have to be discrete. Before I write about actual happenings I need to convey my views as to why Dan had behaved the way he did. I believe that when I was ill in Plymouth he gave me his 100% love and support. This is pretty good going considering I had been unfaithful to him shortly before that. Maybe a lesser man would have turned his back on me. I think by the time we'd reached the St James era Dan was on his last legs and didn't have any more to give, he was emotionally spent. Also there was the apparent likelihood that I would make only a restricted recovery let alone a full one, which must have been both frightening and frustrating. So please keep all of this in mind. I think the main word here would be frustrated, as that was how Dan came across to others and myself. He would treat me badly, be intolerant and behave horribly towards me; but now I can only imagine that was his anger towards the whole situation rather then just me. Our relationship was very strained, with him giving very little support and the marriage often resembled a roller coaster. I guess he was trying to help in a distorted way but his communications and actions were those of a bully and he frequently lost his temper with me. This section is from the notes made by my CPN: ' The relationship between her and her husband is very strained and Lorraine describes feeling 'unloved'.

She finds it difficult talking to him and expressing her feelings, as she states he will not talk about how he feels. Dan has declined to go to Relate with her... she told him, if this 'carries on' she will want to divorce him. She states he appeared not to take her seriously.'

Due to my over medication I was incontinent of urine which happened on a regular occurrence. However on one particular night Dan wouldn't let me change the sheets so I had to lie in my urine for the remainder of the night. Not only was this physically uncomfortable but also mentally degrading and just lowered my self-esteem even further. He just seemed to have zero tolerance for any part of my illness. There were also two other events that were similar to each other which occurred at night and these both left me drowning in a void. Dan was drinking two bottles of wine just about every night; I think this was his way of dealing with the stress. He was drunk, came to bed after me and decided he wanted to be physically gratified; after all I was his wife so in that sense his property. The next day I was the canvas to numerous bruises, but what was more damaged was my mind and soul. I had trusted him, but as I had such a low opinion of myself any way, I felt guilty and regarded myself as a piece of dirt on the floor.

So how have we moved beyond this? Firstly it hasn't been discussed and instead has been meticulously swept under the carpet, in fact I don't know if he even remembers those nights. Secondly for me I know that wasn't the real Dan. He was under so much pressure and had been through such an intolerable degree of pain, how could he be the man that I'd fallen in love with and married? A professional person has recently told me that bipolar individuals can often end up being abused throughout their lives. I guess my life fits in perfectly with that theory. I think now we are constantly growing, moving beyond the illness and building on our sound foundations. So I guess that is the reason why this relationship works and will continue to do so.

During these months it also became very apparent that my mental health problems were exacerbated around the time of my periods. I think that as my condition improved and I started getting more good days, the premenstrual syndrome symptoms stood out. I was referred to a Gynaecologist again with the view to having a hysterectomy. However at our consultation the doctor wanted further medical evidence that this was the actual situation and that I would also be able to tolerate the HRT. I was very disappointed with this decision as basically I was desperate to do anything that would improve my condition. This meant going back on the Zoladex injections combined with HRT. I have now been on this regime for over a year, as I mentioned in an earlier chapter. The benefits are obvious from a medical viewpoint (and mine for that matter!). I am currently waiting for an operation to remove my ovaries, which will mean no more 'horse' injections (the needle that is used for the Zoladex injection is huge!). I will have to continue with the HRT but that is a small price to pay if it means avoiding those dramatic hormonal mood swings.

Now I shall discuss the therapy that I have received. I started seeing a Cognitive Behaviour Therapist who I built a great rapport with and I still see him to this day. I can really relate to this type of therapy and it has helped me greatly. The one thing I really appreciate is that not once did this therapist give up on me, even when I was so profoundly over medicated. I need to make this clear for a particular reason that you will discover shortly. I also started seeing Lisa a therapist who specialized in CAT. Virtually from the onset I had problems relating and trusting her. In this relationship there was no rapport between us. When Lisa stopped seeing me she informed another professional that I was beyond help and should spend the rest of my life in care. Boy would I like to see her now!

This next section is likely to be quite lengthy, as it will consist of my responses to a letter Lisa wrote to my consultant. This to a degree is selfish of me as I'm writing it because I need to have my say, which is something I never achieved at the time. The letter is headed with 'Confidential: not to be seen by patient' and is printed in large bold type. Out of all of my medical notes and letters that I have read for the purpose of this book I have not come across such a statement before. So why was I not meant to read it? I think the reason will soon become apparent to you. To start with she complains about my level of sedation which I guess is reasonable, however my other therapist never stopped seeing me because of my level of sedation, instead I received support and encouragement which wouldn't have gone amiss from her. Lisa then complains of my ambivalent presentation in therapy, giving an example that I would talk about my abusive father but then I would not want to say any more as I would have to get on with my parents. Surely this is logical as my emotional state was very fragile and I was dependent on my parents for support and care. I was not strong enough to deal with the outcome of this issue and could have ended up even more isolated and at risk to myself. Maybe she should have been more constructively supportive and guided me in ways to deal with such conflicts and emotional outcomes.

Lisa also states that I complained of Dan being critical and of his rejection, which crushed my confidence, but then I had told her that my marriage was quite strong and not central to my problems. As I see it marriages fluctuate and that I was unlikely to rock our fragile foundations we had established. Also despite all the difficulties we had experienced our marriage remained intact, which could actually mean it was quite strong and not central to my problems. She also suggests that my ambivalence reflects real dilemmas in my life but I can't discuss them in an honest or open way. Now I wonder if that could actually be down to her, as in the past and present I had built very successful therapeutic relationships without any problems. Maybe it was a fact that I wasn't honest or open because she did not display either of these qualities within the therapeutic relationship.

The next statement cracks me up as she says the only comfortable role I can occupy is 'as someone depressed/needy/helpless (and trying to cope).' I can't help wondering what this means as it seems very contradictory. She implies that I can only display a helpless role but then in brackets I'm trying to cope! Does this mean that my attempts were too futile and pathetic to acknowledge; or that the reality of me trying doesn't fit into her description of me being helpless etc. Maybe I was only comfortable in that role because it was all I knew and all I could possibly be. Lisa also raises the point that I frequently contacted the service feeling suicidal. I can't see this being a problem as that is partly what the service is for. AST especially have managed to stop me from attempting suicide on numerous occasions, as they have provided the support that I greatly needed. Lisa writes that when she addressed this subject I was defensive and claimed that I was misunderstood. Maybe it was Lisa's approach that elicited my anger and defence mechanisms, so when I claimed that I was misunderstood I actually meant by her.

In a long-winded way Lisa claims I was being two faced, saying one thing to her and something completely different to another. She appears more centred on the fact that I could actually be doing that to her rather then the reasons behind it. I think one needs to remember (as she pointed out) I was on heavy medication so my thoughts would obviously be confused at times whilst my memory was impaired, hence saying different things to different people. Surely it would have been of a greater benefit to address this issue, whilst providing support and discovering solutions or new appropriate ways of thinking. This then gets even more confusing as she states that at a later appointment these issues were discussed openly by me, so where was the problem?   Lisa also hints that the reason I dropped out of her therapy was because I was unable to set goals for change, as the two coincided. The reality of the situation was that I had been unhappy with both the therapy and relationship for a while. I discussed these issues with a number of people and after much thought accompanied with advice I decided to end the therapy. She also said that her work clarified the situation. I can't see how it could have done unless she meant highlighting me as a 'bad' client who didn't fit into her expectations.

Well I'm sorry this list seems to be going on forever but I have needed to illustrate this ridiculous 'partnership'! The next point is that I was apparently avoidant of negative emotions. What I would like to know is, who isn't? I will avoid these types of emotions regardless of my mental state; maybe it's a case of the survival of the fittest and the fight or flight syndrome. All I know is that if the more I exposed myself or the more indulgent I became to these emotions then the depression would flow deeper and more turbulently and this is when I would be more likely to make a suicidal attempt. Lisa also makes a point that I depended on medication to suppress my feelings. When I started on these drugs I was in hospital and had no other skills to deal with the distressing feelings apart from self-harm and suicide and as already mentioned I soon became addicted to them. I wonder if she has ever experienced such soul destroying feelings, I think not as there was no degree of sympathy let alone empathy, or she would have understood the medication issues.

We're getting there honest! The next point was made about my threatened suicides, the attempts and the alcohol. My consultant already knew these facts so why was there a need to state it, which seemed more of a complaint then anything else. These actions were the only solutions I had to a bloody awful existence and as far as I'm concerned they reflected the agony of my inner soul. Lisa also said I had extreme anger which I 'disavow' but I act in a passive aggressive manner. I just don't know what to say to this comment; it seems like too many words without any meaning that again contradict each other. However is there any wonder as to why I was angry? She also believed my problems were: 'a complex phenomenon and not (ONLY) a biological illness'. Again this was stating the obvious for all concerned, so what was the point? At times I think she had no idea of my past history or why would she make such unoriginal 'revelations'. Lisa also wrote that I had a personality disorder. This is a very serious diagnosis to make which can have many repercussions and I find it quite irresponsible of her considering how little she knew of me as a person. Having such a disorder can make treatment complicated and my current psychiatrist has said that although I have an impulsive personality I definitely do not have a disorder. I know whom I have the confidence to believe. I just wonder what damage she could have made to my treatment if this label had stuck for any amount of time.

Three more issues to go! This next one is about the role I had incorporated of being 'ill with depression' within a range of 'Dysfunctional interpersonal procedures'. What other role would I have had, as I'd recently been discharged for a depressive illness after thirteen months in hospital? In this situation I would imagine that everyone's personal interactions were not functioning correctly. Again I can't understand why she used all this jargon to start with, but then she writes as though she's informing my psychiatrist of a revolutionary finding.

In summary Lisa felt I wasn't suitable for any therapy at that time, and certainly not CAT in the near or distant future. So how did I manage to get on so well with CAT in Plymouth, and why was I progressing well with CBT at that time? Finally it came across that Lisa was leaving a sinking ship and by 'relinquishing my challenging care' she could only 'help indirectly', so by Lisa doing this I confidently presume that she deemed no hope for me and was getting out early so I couldn't be classified as one of her failures. In a way I would say she had no anticipation of a recovery for me in any shape or form. After I informed her that I would not be continuing with these sessions I received a letter from her telling me she knew that I was keen to manage my problems and that she was confident I could build upon the changes I had begun. To me this is a contradiction to the official 'secret' letter I have just dissected. As far as I'm concerned in view of all the evidence it was a case of the rat leaving the sinking ship.

I feel one of the most important aspects of therapy is the relationship between the therapist and client. If there appears to be no rapport, you don't trust them or have a bad 'gut' feeling then don't pursue with the therapy as very little will be gained from it. Just because a person has a title after their name it does not mean that they are without question skilled. As in all walks of life there are individuals who are good and others that are bad at their profession. Or it could easily be a case of personalities clashing. I think my major belief is to feel empowered in that you are able to take control and remain an active part of the therapeutic relationship rather then a passive one. A person needs to remember that despite having problems or being ill, they have the given right to freedom of choice so should actively use it. As for the professionals I think they need to remember that the client can be vulnerable, nervous and often wary. A display of genuine empathy, understanding and above all respect needs to be shown. We are all different people, with varying pasts and changing needs and not just a medical label. I believe ultimately therapy should be based on trust and honesty for both parts of the equation.

As I've already mentioned my mood was still dismal and fluctuating until February/March 2003. I believe my consultant (Dr Ash) took a great gamble with me at times, for which I am eternally grateful to him. There were many outpatient appointments when I was extremely suicidal and displayed a whole array of severely depressive symptoms. He strongly believed (and I presume even more so in my case) that hospitalization institutionalized and deskilled people, so he took the risk of keeping me in the community, which paid off. It must have been so disheartening and frustrating that week after week there would be no change in my condition. During the worst patches my consultant saw me more frequently and regularly. He is another person who never gave up on me and I believed in him at that time. In hindsight I feel frustrated that I wasn't given the correct diagnosis and therefore the treatment and drugs I so desperately need. So here we are again with the same old repetitive feature. I can't change the past and what will be will be.

Although this next part officially crosses over to the following chapter I would like to include it here. This is basically a summary of my last meeting with

Dr Ash and therefore my discharge back to my GP. (I do want to add here that I will be discussing my excellent GP in my final chapter.) In my GP's letter Dr Ash describes my recovery as remarkable and that I stated I had no mental health symptoms. I also described to him that my family life was good and that I was coping well with the children. I actually took them along to that appointment and they burst into cascades of uncontrollable giggles, which also triggered off Dr Ash and myself! He described to the GP how very happy the children were. The rest of the session was spent discussing my relapse risk (around 50-60% but not as severe – oh joy of joys), the further reduction of medication that could take place and the frequency of the blood tests that were needed. Eventually I was discharged and about time to! The only cloud on this horizon was the fact that I wasn't remarkably well at all. Instead the reality was that I had entered a hypomanic state, so it was more a case of the individual wave couldn't be seen due to the vastness of the sea. I watched the sunrise and headed off to manic waters.

CHAPTER TWELVE – ENDING THE PASSAGE AT IT'S START

Apart from vague disjointed memories of Christmas and New Year of 2002/2003, my next or should I say first, clear and exact memories are of March 2003. I can remember this time, as I was quite physically unwell. This involved numerous trips to the GP with an equal amount of diagnosis. Dan was actually at sea and I can remember trying desperately hard to get him home. This is something I haven't even contemplated in the past year, despite everything. My final diagnosis was an excessive level of Liothyronine (one of my drugs) in my body, which matched all of my symptoms. Our au pair went home for Easter and Dan had 2 weeks leave. During this time, we also discovered that we were moving to a larger house locally, which would mean a fresh start for all of us. Through spending time as a family I rediscovered life. I learnt how to laugh again and once I started I couldn't stop! I discovered that I had two fantastic, caring (albeit cheeky) children and this was a wonderful revelation to me. One of the greatest comments Dan made to me over this holiday was: "it's so lovely to be able to laugh with you again Lorry". I guess there must have been a glimmer of hope for him that I was coming back. This joyous period was soon over, so it was time to collect the au pair and for Dan to return to Plymouth. Something had happened to me, my determination, fight and spirit had returned at long last. Once I make my mind up about something, I become dedicated to the cause. This time, the cause would be my return to health and life.

My energy started to creep back, along with my strength of mind and my independence started to grow again. I also became determined to lose the remaining 4 stone that I had put on in hospital. I'm not saying it was easy, in fact it was far from that and I did have very difficult moments when suicide became the main item on my agenda. One example of this is when I did my disappearing act at two in the morning whilst extremely drunk. After some bizarre phone calls Sue came round to check things out and found both my tablets and me missing. She called the Police and they went out looking for me, but luckily it was Sue who picked me up and we headed off to the sea for some soul searching. I must highlight that I did survive and every achievement meant a stride in the right direction.

Around about this time I was also offered a total hysterectomy, to finally eradicate the hormonal problems that had strong links to my 'clinical depression'. Just for a bit of background knowledge, we had to really push to get this operation, as I was unusually young for it and without physiological reasons. I'm not sure what happened or even when I decided, but suddenly I knew things had to change. The return of our au pair had been suffocating me. I just wanted to be a mother again in my own right and I wanted to move into our new home as just the four of us, so we could have a fresh start. It didn't take me long to find a solution. I did not to go ahead with the hysterectomy.

I knew I wanted the au pair to leave and the only way I could justify this and therefore make it happen was not to have the operation. Although this meant carrying on with the 12 weekly injections (the equivalent of a drug induced hysterectomy) it was a small price to pay. I ran it past Mum and she supportively said it was my body and therefore my choice. Dan was more wary and concerned that I wouldn't manage on my own, but I was determined and I gave him very little room to manoeuvre. As always I had to get everything done 'yesterday', so I decided to tell the au pair that evening, when she returned from college. She took it well once I'd given reassurance that it wasn't her fault and we would continue to give support until she found a different position. However once I'd told her, I just felt desperate to have my home and space back. Luckily her boyfriend was due the following day, so the children and I stayed at my parents, thus giving us all time and space to think. I'm not religious but I actually prayed that whole weekend for her to return to Czechoslovakia. I just felt one more day with them here, was one day too much. When we returned on the Sunday she informed me that she would be leaving with her boyfriend. I could have shouted with delight and freedom. The next couple of days were uncomfortable between us, especially as her boyfriend's behaviour was so unimpressive. We told the children together the following night expecting them to be upset. At times I think children can be so misjudged. Their only concerns were who would be looking after them and once they knew it would be me, they were more then happy with the situation.

We had three au pairs in total, the last being the best, but once she'd gone all sorts of tales were springing forth from various people. Two of who were the children, they independently and voluntarily told me how the second au pair used to 'pull their pants down and hit them lots.' This not only horrifies me but also breaks my heart. To think that we welcomed this person into our home; that we had mistakenly trusted her and she had hit our children on a regular basis. We don't even hit our children; it is viewed as an extreme last resort, let alone someone else doing it. From that time onwards, no matter what, I have promised that I will never, ever have another au pair under my roof. Especially when combining this with the many other situations we have since been informed about.

I think that when our third au pair left us, I entered a full blown hypomanic state, where as before that there was only just a hint of it. Suddenly I had so much energy, an alien feeling to me, I literally did not know what to do with it all. I would stay up until 1am, go to bed and then get up at 4am, whilst the whole time I was awake I would be active. My aim at that point was to sort out the entire rubbish ready for our move, less than a few weeks away. In fewer than five days I turned out more than 40 bags full of 'rubbish', most of which went to charity shops. I was completely reckless in my sorting, this included anyone's belongings that I hadn't seen or used in the past 3 years. Naturally this amounted to an awful lot considering I had been a zombie for the majority of that time. Also anything that had the slightest hint of my illness, or of the au pairs, I threw away. One thing that horrified me during this time was the dirt and filth that covered our home. This was meant to be another of the au pair's jobs, yet it was disgusting. I had always taken care in maintaining our home, so this was a repulsive shock to actually realize the state we had been living in.

During this week I ate next to nothing, overflowed with energy, regained confidence with driving, and rediscovered shopping. I also became extremely sociable, something that had obviously been missing over the previous years. Various family members and friends warned me to slow down, but as far as I could make out I was fine, in fact more then fine. I even told my CPN (when she visited) exactly what I had been up to and the way I'd been behaving, but she obviously didn't see a problem so therefore I couldn't see a reason to worry or stop.

We moved house and as Dan had been away a lot I did nearly all of the organising and sorting out. Although I got tired during the move I quickly bounced back. I seemed to be in my element looking after the house and kids, doing all the shopping, cleaning, and ironing. I had gone from vegetating in a chair to being 100% active in a matter of days. When I woke up at 4am I would get up and start my chores and anything else that I could find to do, such as taking down and cleaning all of the curtains. Goodness knows what the neighbors must have thought if they'd seen me doing these activities at such an early time in the morning. My psychiatrist also discharged me at this point. I do wonder how he didn't recognize this behaviour for what it was, i.e. hypomania. Maybe he was just really pleased but at the same time relieved that I was 'cured' and he didn't want to or have the time to delve any deeper. However he was a decent man so I expect it was the case that it never even occurred to him, after all Bipolar Disorder is difficult to diagnose.

My passionate affair with shopping also began around about this time. It gave me such a buzz and I could not stop or prevent myself from spending, even if it was just the weekly food shop. On the rare occasions that I did finally sit down, I would spend ages looking through home shopping catalogues and this soon became my favourite, relaxing past time. In total I spent about £4,000, something that we now have to deal with. We also purchased a new car and I went from a wary driver to an extremely confident one and although I stayed within the legal limits I became a fast driver. This would also give me a rush of adrenaline and the excitement that I craved. Confidence just oozed out of me, I was always extremely friendly, knew just the right thing to say, made appropriate and witty jokes and I always seemed to be organizing others. I also lost 3 stone during this time and although I started off dieting, I soon discovered that I didn't have to, as the weight just carried on dropping off me. The summer was fantastic for the kids and they fondly (I hasten to add) call it 'Mummy's crazy time'! If we weren't up to at least 3 activities or outings a day, then something was seriously wrong. This meant they certainly got tired and went to bed early, which unfortunately gave me more time to drink. Although my alcohol consumption crept up, I just didn't seem to get hangovers and was able to tolerate much larger quantities. The drinking just accelerated my good mood without slowing me down. On the sexual side I just wasn't able to get enough. After being abstinent for so long during my depression this increased desire was great, but I always had this impression that I was some sort of sex 'goddess' with tempting sexual abilities.

The last issue that I can poignantly remember was being 'looked after' by some higher force. This was independent of my lack of religious beliefs, however I felt that I was always being guided to make the best choices and that life would always turn out for the right reasons just because... It was almost like gambling, placing a bet on my 'guided' choice, yet I would always come up winning. This was how all my decisions were made, whether it was something as simple as what I would eat to big life changing behaviours. My luck of always being right seemed to stay with me, until the depression set in, stealing it all away from my desperate and grasping hands.

My Cognitive Behavioural Psychologist of that time (and still remains so) was a brilliant man and he has helped me immensely. He never gave up on me, even at my bleakest times, when others had condemned me to spending the remainder of my life in care. I always left our sessions with a different view of how to tackle my problems, a clearer mind to see with and ultimately armed with a greater knowledge and understanding. However I decided the time was right to stop seeing him. Sensibly he didn't break all ties and thankfully left his door open for me in the future. When I think back, I realize that I kept a lot of these hypomanic behaviours and thoughts from him, albeit subconsciously. It was almost as though, at some level I was aware that something was wrong, but the way I felt was just too good to surrender. Relatives and friends say now that I was always gushing my words and talking too much. I knew my brain was constantly on the go, but to be honest it was just fantastic to have a brain again. I guess the gift of hindsight is an interesting one, but despite the possible future value, it is of very little use in healing the past. At this present time I am pleased to say that I am back to my regular appointments with my therapist, which I greatly appreciate. I regard these as a continual lifeline. I know that without them I would surely drown.

Finally at the end of the summer, I had a really weird 24hrs. My brain was racing so fast; I had absolutely no chance to catch up with it. The experience is difficult to describe but I'll try: if you imagine a tape recorder with just your voice on it and then someone (out of your control) presses the fast forward button, leaving you unable to catch up with the words as they are constantly just out of your reach. I was also fully aware that I knew exactly what my movements were at least 10 paces before they happened. I phoned Mum as she was in Cornwall and I told her that something weird was happening to me, she reassured me that I was probably just stressed. Well that was fine by me, although I must admit I was scared. It's strange though, as it was almost as if I knew, because I described myself at the time as being manic.

Progressively and slowly things started to go back down. I kept wondering what was wrong because I wasn't feeling the 'normal' high, but I didn't stop at a base rate instead I kept on going. To start with it was a few days at a time and was blamed on all manner of things from HRT to Lithium levels. Until eventually in October I was back down in a depression, something I emphatically denied, as I couldn't accept the reality of it. I eventually saw my wonderful GP and before I knew it I was potentially admitted to the private psychiatric hospital. I stopped these arrangements mid flow, but agreed to an out patient appointment with one of the psychiatrists. I only saw him a few times and I wasn't fully aware then, but he was the doctor that had handed me over to the NHS on my return from Plymouth. I knew there must have been a reason as to why I wasn't comfortable with him. He suggested on each occasion that I should go into hospital, but I always refused due to my horrendous NHS experience. My Lithium was increased, I was told to sort out my own a antidepressant medication, that I had to face up to things and accept my diagnosis and that I would 'have to agree to a CPN referral', to which I completely refused. I just decided I wasn't accepting it and there was no way I was going back under NHS care via a CPN. Thank goodness my psychologist (I was seeing him again) was brilliantly supportive and he suggested that I went for a second opinion with a consultant psychiatrist that he recommended.

I didn't rush as my depression had lifted, but on reflection I can now recognize that I was creeping above 'normal' again. My husband was returning from sea (after 3 months away) and it was going to be our first proper Christmas in 4 years, one that I would actually remember. Maybe the excitement just propelled me up again, as my spending had got completely out of hand, I was constantly organizing and rushing around and I couldn't stop talking. Also since I'd got depressed in the autumn I was drinking every night, at least a bottle and a half of wine. Over the Christmas period my consumption just kept on going up, with spirits and lager added to the equation. I would just think 'never mind it is Christmas'. I think I must have gone over the top during the first week of the New Year. We'd gone away to a farmer's cottage in

Somerset. I seemed obsessed with being organized and getting my point of view across. The words were pouring from my mouth and I was coming out with sentences obviously before I had given them any thought. Hence they often had very little meaning and at times were very offensive. When we returned home the house was an absolute mess and Dan returned to Plymouth. I didn't stop again, it was as though some inner force drove me and my drinking continued every night.

The appointment for my second opinion had arrived and I attended it with Sue for moral support. This time I was impressed (unlike before) straight away as this man had an amazing peace, calm and knowledge about him. I instantly trusted and liked him; but I also knew I had to be completely honest because it didn't feel as though he'd accept any bullshit from me! After half an hour of asking me questions he confidently gave me a diagnosis of Bipolar Disorder. "Isn't that manic depression?" I quietly asked, only to already know that the answer was yes. It made complete sense but I couldn't believe it, I was in shock. After all I hadn't expected a new diagnosis, instead I'd only wanted to hear that my depression could be resolved. I knew this was a life long condition, with no cure as yet and that meant medication for the rest of my life. I think I must have gone numb for a few days. I did go straight home that night and drank, despite being unquestionably told not to by the consultant. Alcohol was my crutch, my friend and my enemy. I did have a basic knowledge of this condition, but people around me were saying it makes no difference and they all just seemed too busy to hear my pain and confusion. I knew in my heart, even if not in my brain at this point, that this was indeed very different. Alongside this the normal cycle was taking place; so following the Christmas high I entered a depression, this one being more stubborn and deeper than the last.

At the same time my sister had her delayed wedding dinner and dance. I was confronted with 160 people, lots of alcohol and loads of stress. I think that when I applied my make up that night I also painted a smile on to greet all the comments such as: "You look so well, don't let yourself go down again, wasn't that an awful time for your family (I wouldn't know I couldn't be there), keep this up." It's hard work dealing with this for 5 hours when inside you're screaming, "no it's not ok, I want to kill myself and as an added bonus ball I have Bipolar Disorder which is a life long sentence!" My mind had many more comments stored up but I don't want this to be full of bad language. I guess without surprise, I got completely and utterly drunk, knocking the alcohol back until 4am. The next day extremely and revoltingly hung over, I tackled the book of Patty Duke's life with Bipolar Disorder. This at least was a start, I recognized myself in her words, but I still couldn't quite accept it.

My depression deepened, with all the symptoms mentioned in chapter one to varying degrees and I could barely function. I saw my GP and my appointment was brought forward by my consultant. During this time when I saw him or my therapist, I found that I could sit completely silent for a few moments. This allowed my mind to be still enough so that I didn't have to put up the constant struggle against the suicidal thoughts and in a way it was peaceful. I was not sleeping, so was extremely tired,

I was not eating but instead drinking heavily. So let alone mentally I was also a wreck physically, hence it was pretty apparent I would have to be admitted. Although I didn't agree immediately I wasn't as stubborn as before. I think this was purely down to my consultant as I actually trusted him and his direction was so quiet and peaceful there seemed to be no effort. It was just a case of me saying yes that's the route I have to take and although it felt like my decision I knew it had been his.

When I informed people of my impending admission I received a lot of opposition. I know it was because of their own fears due to the past NHS experience, but I just felt like I barely had the energy to keep alive, let alone relay their concerns as well. I was heartbroken when I said goodbye to my children. It seems crazy now but all I could think of, was what type of state would I be in when I see them next. I'm sure in their own simplistic way, they were having the same thoughts. It may also seem mad, but it was a hard wrench leaving our puppy, as I'd put so much time and effort into training her. Whilst over the previous few weeks, even more so then normal, she had been a fantastic companion showing me unconditional love no matter how I was feeling. I was terrified when I went in, although Dan was supportive and attempted to maintain my humour. My consultant asked me if there was any other reason, apart from the obvious, as to why I would be so scared. At the time I couldn't think, but I do know now, it was because my daughter's birth had been so soul destroying and yet again involved a hospital admission. I guess it was no surprise that I had so little trust in such establishments, I just didn't want to relinquish my control.

I'm not going to analyze this hospital admission to pieces; yet again I'm going to pull out parts that were important to me. After my first night, I was in so much psychological pain and so obsessed with suicidal thoughts that I felt out of control. I wasn't any good at saying how I felt or asking for help, hence the next situation occurred. I sat in my chair, with my back to the door, looking out of the window. I felt numb in one instant and the next as if I wanted to scream and howl. All I really knew was that I desperately wanted to die; I needed peace and for everything to be over. Nothing else mattered. I know I was building up to this, as I told my therapist the previous week that I'd reached the stage at which I needed to self-harm again. I started biting my left hand really hard, at first I could feel pain but that soon stopped. My mind frantically evaluated what I could use to cause greater pain and then I realized I had my mobile phone. I timed it so that I could hit myself after the nurse had just been in to check me (I was on 10 minute observations) and then I knew I had 10 clear minutes alone until the next check. I kept furiously hitting the phone onto the back of my hand. I've no idea how long I kept this up for, but I was compelled to carry on, it was something I just had to keep on doing. I suspect you could classify this as obsessive, however the release of pain was absorbing. First of all there was a small swelling on the back of my hand and then gradually it was completely swollen up like a balloon. As I smashed my hand more and more it became agonizing. I had to bite hold of my top to stop myself from yelling out and after each attack (always 5 hits but I don't know why), I'd quickly smoke a fag to fight off the waves of nausea and pain. Despite all of this pain it actually felt calming psychologically; that deep absorbing agony that had infiltrated my mind had a release. Just like turning the controls on a pressure cooker releasing the steam (pain). I couldn't find the words to describe the mental anguish, but this act of physical pain said many to me and psychologically I felt better.

It wasn't long before my fingers, hand and wrist were swollen completely; somehow I had to make myself stop. I didn't want to end up with broken bones, a plaster cast and therefore a physical show for all to see. I knew the only way to stop, as I'd gone too far and was now out of control, was to tell someone. I refused to go to Casualty, insisting that I hadn't broken it. The next day I didn't have any choice, my hand was even more swollen, it was starting to turn black and I had red tracts travelling up my arm. It wasn't broken, but was infected so I needed a sling and two types of antibiotics. I cringed at this, as the whole thing was now on public display. Something that originally was an extremely private action was now available for all to see. I didn't want it shouted out to everyone that I was in such mental anguish, but now I had no choice. This was so similar to the past, where I never saw beyond the act of causing harm or what the following consequences would be. I actually felt worse after this. I am still having problems with it now.

Now with my logical, healthy head screwed on I realize how wrong and terribly distressing that way of thinking is. I did make another attempt the following weekend this time with the toilet roll holder (I was running out of dangerous weapons) and my right hand. I did cut it enough to draw blood (and I still have the scar), but after a few attempts I thought "hang on, you need help." This time

I actually managed to ask for it, before things went too far. Perhaps the therapy was helping after all. The following week my mind was fully occupied with a course about Cognitive Behavior Therapy on self-harm and suicidal thoughts. This involved studying from a book in my room alone. I could really relate to the literature and not only did I understand it, I gained greatly by expressing myself through writing and I actually took it all on board.

Later in that week I became possessed by suicidal and self harm demons once again. This was a torturous walk through hell. By this stage I was not allowed any extra medication to help me. I sat facing the window silently screaming inside, shaking, crying and became a heap of emotional distress. This time I chose to tell the staff and to talk with them. I received an awful lot of support and understanding. Between us I got through it, but I had to use the skills I had just learnt and a lot of determination. I still felt shaken and that I was a failure until the inpatient therapist came to see me. He actually showed me how to turn my thoughts around and helped me realize a lot of things mainly about my own strengths. My feelings on this can be found in the concluding chapter.

So I've nearly reached the point where I started, sitting in this hospital chair. Since then I have been up for a couple of days and then down for a couple of days, although definitely not depressed and I believe my new medication regime is certainly having a positive effect. I'm just waiting for a few more days to ensure that I'm stable. Hopefully by then I will be discharged, back with my children and dog (Dan's at sea), a place where I long to be. So this is a grand total of four and a half weeks, rather different from thirteen months. I do sometimes sit here wondering what if? What if I'd come here instead of St James? Then I expect the past few years would have been different. However what has happened has happened and I can't bring it back or change it. I certainly don't believe that these experiences have made me the person I am, I have always been that person but just changing slightly as time flows past. What I can do is be thankful for the here and now, for having such a fantastic team supporting me and for having my mental health at this moment in time. I'm not sure what lies ahead, but then no one does. Although with the professional support I have, I feel confident that I will get through anything, riding the waves of the highs and lows. Watch this space this yacht is sailing places!

CHAPTER THIRTEEN – REFLECTIONS OF A TRANQUIL SEA

I started to write this chapter whilst I was in hospital however at that moment in time I had no idea how vast this book would turn out to be. I will include my thoughts from that period but they will flow alongside my impressions since completing this work. I regarded the private hospital to be an asylum in the correct sense of the word i.e. a refuge or sanctuary. Whilst I was there I gained a number of invaluable gifts. To begin with I was provided with protection from my own mind when it was sick, thus allowing me to rest and recharge my batteries in a safe harbour. I was also provided with priceless tools that have enabled me to live a healthy and as normal a life as possible. This has been accomplished not only via the support of the nursing staff and general therapists, but also through my consultant and the cognitive behaviour techniques that my in-patient therapist Adam taught me. This man was a larger than life character, full of energy and enthusiasm. I think most importantly for me it was the skills he had in challenging my thoughts with such ease. He was able to completely turn around my unhealthy and destructive beliefs, which ultimately led to a robust way of thinking. His influence on me is still apparent now and I use the skills he taught me throughout my daily life.

I also need to express my deepest gratitude to my consultant not only for the time he took to listen and share ideas with me, but also for finally sorting out my biochemical imbalances and restoring me to a whole and functioning individual. Without his skills, expertise and wisdom I would not be sitting here now feeling happy and peaceful. At my very worst times when I was battling with the suicidal demons but without the 'help' of any drugs, it would feel as though Adam was on one of my shoulders and my consultant on the other as if they were two good spirits willing me on. The entire time I felt that I couldn't let them down as they had put so much time and effort in to my care and belief into my being. I knew absolutely that I could not fail them, so I kept on fighting and pulled through the nightmare.

The key word to extract from all of this is hope. Adam taught me that with hope it is possible to achieve anything. For the suicidal person it's having the hope that the future will get better and if this is truly believed then the suicidal thoughts will become quiet until they are no longer heard. Another example for me is to have the hope that the agitation will dissolve and consequently the self-harm desires fade. Basically it's simply to have hope for your future.

Two other facts that Adam highlighted to me were that firstly the reason I couldn't stimulate my own recovery in St James' was because I was so over medicated. I had always believed it was something I had done wrong and that I had been extremely weak, as a result of this I had been carrying around a lot of guilt on my shoulders. Adam concluded for me that if I didn't rely on drugs I would be able to fight for my own survival. From this he also illustrated the fact that during my worst time in the private hospital I was able to get through it on my own determination and without the use of medication. Both these points made me feel that I could have belief and faith in myself, which automatically provides me with hope for my future. Through Cognitive Behavioural Therapy I learnt how to deal with the destructive thoughts involved in anxiety, depression, agitation, self-harm and suicide. Being armed with these new skills and having methods to manage the negative thoughts I discovered I had an all-empowering feeling of hope for the future. I use these skills every day and when faced with a problem I think through what I have been taught so that I can adapt it to the situation.

I now work with my long-standing Cognitive Behavioural therapist and as I have mentioned before I can't begin to stress the help and encouragement he has given me. Especially the fact that throughout our therapeutic relationship he has never given up on me. The last person I need to mention from the medical team that supports me is my GP. He has always been there for me, agreeing to see me at a moments notice, phoning me at home if he has results or I have concerns. He has always shown genuine empathy and an understanding of my situation. When I was first diagnosed with Bipolar Disorder he was fantastic. On the day of my 'second opinion' he made it clear that I could see him the following day if I needed to. So it goes without saying that I took him up on the offer albeit at the last moment. I sat in his office and cried for about forty minutes. Throughout that time he reassured me, helped me to become aware of the positives and told me of success stories as well as looking up information on the Internet. What I really remember though is that he held my hand and just let me cry until there were no more tears to shed. As you can see I have a fantastic medical team behind me and I can see hope for my future. I now know that I'm equipped with skills to challenge all that is thrown at me, and if this is not enough I have the back up of an outstanding medical team, so the only path I need to follow is that of hope; whilst trying my hardest not to lose touch of it when I become ill again.

Well I guess this really brings me on to how I feel about my bipolar diagnosis. The point, at which I'm now at, is one where I think I've accepted it and I'm even glad to have the label (not the illness though!). At least now I have the correct diagnosis so the treatment can be modified to manage the illness. At the start of this book I wanted to cry every time I thought about it. Sometimes I still whisper, "why me?" I just think I need to live my life and get on with it. However I find myself being very reluctant to tell people about my condition now. This book does not have a happy ending though, as I live my life in the shadow of this illness. I never know when I will become ill again and if it will manifest itself in the form of hypomania or depression.

There are methods that I've had to learn in an attempt to maintain equilibrium. Such examples are as simple as leaving caffeine out of my diet and promoting sleep; to structuring my life style and managing stress and conflict more efficiently. A really big issue is the taking of medications correctly and on time. I am currently on ten different drugs and I have to take a combination of these twice a day, so I have resorted to using a pillbox otherwise I wouldn't manage it. Also I need to monitor my mood on a frequent basis and if I notice the same abnormal state on more then three consecutive days I have to get in touch with my consultant. In conjunction with these methods I have to have regular blood tests carried out. I think one of my most frustrating daily experiences is when I'm tired or exposed to excess external stimuli. At these times my brain seems to shut down on me, I can't think, I can't concentrate, I can't hear people and I can't make decisions. The hardest part of this is that I'm never aware as to when it will happen instead everything just suddenly stops. I try to be discrete about this problem especially if I'm with people who are unaware of my illness, however at times I have to disappear to a quiet corner until my faculties return and I can continue normally.

I no longer feel angry towards the words Bipolar Disorder, but remnants of that emotion still resound when I think of my past. Through writing this book I think I have a greater understanding as to why such soul destroying experiences have happened to me but that doesn't make them any more just or acceptable; but I know that I need to move on with my thoughts and ultimately with my life. With regards to the echoes of my eating disorder I have stopped weighing myself every day. Instead I have joined a diet club, which is establishing healthy eating practices in my life, with the aim that I will lose my remaining excess weight under a controlled situation. I have started drinking alcohol again, but not to the degree that I was before, especially when I was ill. I'm trying to be sensible by monitoring my intake to maintain it within the recommended allowances and if I don't feel well I don't drink. I didn't join the AA's in the end, I'm not entirely sure why. I couldn't dispel the myth in my head that it was connected to religion and I didn't want to walk into a group of strangers regardless as to whether I had to confess all or not. Don't get me wrong I do think it's a worthwhile organization and the members I spoke to following my discharge seemed great. However for some reason it didn't seem the right time or place for me. I guess this will be an on going issue in my life, but at the moment it is one that I confidently feel I have control over. Maybe I'm wrong, who knows and perhaps I will have to tackle it again further along the horizon. With regards to the hormonal problem, as already mentioned, I am waiting to hear if I can have my ovaries removed which should eradicate it once and for all.

This finally leaves me with the matter of suicide. At the moment I can say 100% that I am not experiencing any suicidal ideations in any shape or form. However I don't know what the future will hold for me but the prospect of suicide has become an alternative option for me and is in a way my safety net. I know if things go dreadfully wrong again I can resort to taking my life and I have a large supply of drugs to enable me to accomplish this goal. If I feel compelled to take such drastic actions I know I will succeed as I have a fool-proof plan and I'm sure that I won't make any mistakes again. This isn't meant to be shocking instead it's honesty and just describes my back up plan (obviously not in detail as I don't want to give anything away), so it's just in case the question 'what if?' arises then I have an answer ready. I do want to strongly add though that I now have hope for my future and I'm not expecting to use such drastic measures.

I have also discovered a method of coping with my impulsive personality. Basically when ever I get a burning thought that I feel desperate to act upon I write it down on paper in detail. I then leave it for an hour or even overnight, after which time I reread it to see if I feel the same urgency and to determine if it is appropriate or not. I will repeat this procedure until I feel that I need to throw the paper and therefore my thoughts, away into the bin or that it is actually ok to go ahead and act upon it. This might seem a bit strange but it is in fact very effective and prevents a lot of 'after the event' embarrassment!

The next areas I need to look at are the relationships in my life. I think I will start with my children. They seem very happy, confident and well adjusted beings. Both of them have an understanding of this illness to a certain degree. They know that when things get too hectic, noisy or racy that Mummy's brain 'switches off'. At this point they understand that they have to sit quietly downstairs, play in their bedrooms or spend their energy in the garden. They have completely grasped the concept of this illness in that I can be 'very, very happy' or 'very, very sad' and they relate this back to my hospital stays and last summer. They know it's not Mummy's fault or anything they've done, but instead it's like Nana's diabetes or when they get a tummy ache. I find their understanding fascinating, as in a simplistic way they have grasped more of the essence of this illness then many adults do. I guess their innocence is responsible for the non-judgmental approach they take towards me. Don't get me wrong this isn't a rosy lined cottage story, as at times it's bloody hard, especially as I'm mostly on my own. What I am trying to convey is that the three of us work together to establish equilibrium in our lives. I can't imagine my life without them and many times it is purely the two children that have kept me going. I hope due to their experiences they will grow into adults that know their own mental status and are more accepting of others with such health problems. I worry that they may develop this illness, but we have the advantage in that we know what symptoms to look out for so can seek and implement treatment quickly. All I can really say now is that they are my precious sunrise and always will be.

My family have been brilliant, having always shown me love and although at times it takes a while, they strive for understanding. Since my Bipolar diagnosis Mum and Sue have read many books on the subject to expand their knowledge. For all of us it has been a steep learning curve but I think we are getting there. Mum and Sue in a 'casual' way automatically monitor my moods, they think I don't know but I can tell by their questions. At times it will be hard because I know I will refuse to hear what they say to me, however I also know they will persevere. It's quite comforting to know they are keeping an eye on me and quite often I use them as a sounding board if I'm not too sure about my moods. I am getting on a lot better with my dad, I don't think we will ever be able to establish the missing bond but at least we are friends again. I have also received a lot of support and encouragement from the remaining members of my family. Additionally I need to acknowledge my two sets of in-laws. They have both been good to me, providing a lot of telephone support, helping with the children and actively seeking out information on Bipolar disorder so that they can grasp a better understanding of it.

This leaves Dan and my closest friend, the latter of whom I haven't mentioned yet. Dan and I are getting on well but countless improvements need to be made. He is away at sea most of the time. Affection, love, companionship and physical aspects need to be worked on to improve the relationship but this is the case for many partnerships. The main fact is that despite every thing we are still together which must speak reams. Somehow we need to improve the bonds and our lives, which will depend on communication. So yet again there is no happy ending instead just an ongoing story with a degree of hopeful anticipation.

I do have a small circle of good friends who I am in touch with on a periodic basis but there is one person that I need to specifically mention and that is my closest friend. I have not mentioned her earlier in this book because I know she would not have wanted to be, however it would have been erroneous of me not to recognize her at all. She has been a huge part of my life since my return from Bath, when we first met. I know our relationship has been two-way, but I want to take this opportunity to thank her. She has been with me every single step of the way. No matter what I've done or how I feel, I have always had her unconditional love and support. When there has been no one else she has picked up the pieces and dried my tears, never judging me even when I've been extremely misguided in my decision making. If I've needed someone to listen to me, or simply wanted to hear another's voice she is there for me, no matter what time of the day or night. As much as anything I cherish her wit and humour. Despite the whole world collapsing around us, we will still end up sharing a lot of laughter together. I don't think I could ever find enough words to express my thanks to her, or how much I value our extremely close friendship.

Well this is scary I'm starting to draw to the end of this passage and to be honest I didn't even expect to get this far. The issue of not reaching my goals and finishing something to its conclusion is a feature of my life now, as there are no longer certainties. No running off into a beautiful sunset full of smiles and no happy ending. I have no idea what the future may hold for me even in a vague way. To begin with I couldn't even see a week ahead and I have only recently been able to make tentative plans towards the following month. The problem is that I'm always wondering as to when I will be ill again and in which form the illness will manifest itself i.e. a high or a low mood. I won't commit myself to anything as I don't know how I will be and I wont make promises to my children. Concrete assumptions are out whilst nervous uncertainties are in. I wake up each day hopeful it will be another good one, but I don't take it for granted that it will be. So I hope but I don't presume, however I have been discharged from hospital for three months now, which is a great achievement. In the back of my mind though, I believe there will be more periods of illness. I hope that it won't be as severe as I'm now armed with many tools to challenge it and of course the support from a wonderful medical team. So each day I look to the new sunrise and I am filled with aspirations that a new day brings a new beginning with new possibilities.

I now need to sum up this book from the viewpoint of how it has helped me and the way I hope it has helped others. One of the main positive experiences for me is that by researching and organizing my medical notes I have been able to fill in the gaps in my elusive memory. I can't begin to express how scary it is to have great, big voids where you have no idea of what has happened or at the best just small fragments of events. Now when people talk about the past four years I'm actually able to say, "yes I know that". It's not so much a memory, although at times the information has triggered a small return, but is more of a case of being aware of something so that you are able to regain control of the situation. I've often learnt that certain people gave me greater help and support then I had given them credit for. It is refreshing to form the whole picture rather then only the shattered splinters that were available to me. What I thought I had established before this book as the truth, wasn't always the real situation. However this can work both ways as I also read things that I thought I had forgotten and situations that I couldn't remember and at times it was extremely distressing.

It has also been harrowing at times to surf through the areas of my past that I clearly remember for example my time in Bath. These are crystal clear to me but they have been locked away tightly in a casket so that I have not had to spend any energy or pain in thinking of them. To sit like this and write I have had to confront these experiences and at moments it has felt as though all the years had been erased and I was actually back there, in time reliving the nightmares. During all of these episodes I have had to work so hard using my newly developed Cognitive Behavioural skills, just to keep me from loosing the plot and preventing the pain that it has caused from entering the other realms of my life. However through writing this I have been able to lay to rest a lot my anger and anguish. It's almost as if I have driven out the pain and am replacing it with a peaceful tranquillity. I have been able to complete the jigsaw of my life, which in turn has provoked a lot of torment, however I do believe I have dealt with it in a healthy and efficient way. This isn't just in relation to my hospital experiences but all that I have written about.

The one message that I have gleamed through all of these chapters is that I am a survivor. Once discovering myself in these circumstances I have gone on to fight my way out even if it has been delayed at times. This shouts to me that I am a strong human being and I don't just give up, which yet again reintroduces the word hope. For me to have carried on working my way back to the real world and to deal with such intolerable circumstances I must have had a degree of hope. This can be said for every chapter from the rapes to the Diazepam abuse. I also believe this is how I've dealt with my Bipolar diagnosis. After comparing the past to this diagnosis I believed my future could not be as painful and traumatic as that. Now I think, at least I have been properly diagnosed so that I can receive the correct treatment, therefore from a logical viewpoint my future cannot be as tormenting as my previous existence. Again I am keeping the word hope close to my side.

Well that's what I have achieved so far, now it's time to cast this over to the flowing seas of the general public. Ideally I hope this will reach the hands of three groups of people: those who are living with mental illness, the professionals treating them and the fortunate individuals who have been lucky enough not to experience it. Firstly I would like to let the individual experiencing such illnesses know that they are not alone and that many people are psychologically challenged every day and from every walk of life. Also that the thoughts they are having are not unusual or strange so it is ok to go and seek professional support. I describe numerous conditions in this book from eating disorders, anxiety and suicidal ideations to mention but a few. Just remember you are not alone in this world and you can get help. I know my story isn't finished but it should give you some hope that life can get better and you have the potential to improve your health. Just try and grasp some hope from these pages and draw it towards your own life.

Secondly my desire was to give a comprehensible account to mental health professionals as to what it's like to actually experience such illnesses. My aim was to create a clearly illustrated picture that would encompass the reader, in the hope that they could feel the suffering rather then just see it as words alone. In this way I aspire to elicit a degree of empathy and understanding that a standard factual textbook could not. If this can be achieved to any degree it will surely help in the treatment and recovery of an individual. I know that the times I have been understood are those when I have responded the greatest and my recovery has been the most efficient; a prime example is that of my recent hospital admission. So surely this has benefits to both sides of the mental health coin.

Finally it would be beneficial if the 'healthy' individual were able to cast their eyes over a few pages. Again the fundamental word here is understanding. If this book were able to educate a person in any of these mental health issues then the spread of such knowledge would be invaluable. Hopefully in this way some of the bias and myths towards people with mental health issues could be diminished, which would lead to an all round, greatly improved society. I guess we can live in hope.

So here I am on my last paragraph of this long passage. I think I only have three key words I need to validate. Firstly is the word HAPPINESS. For me it is waking up with a smile upon my face (or after my first cuppa!), it is a gift in itself that I'm sure anyone who has experienced depression will agree with. Happiness is the glittering crest of a wave. Secondly is the word PEACE. To experience peace of mind and body is food for the soul and should never be taken for granted. My perception of peace is that of a tranquil sea. Finally, is the word HOPE. It automatically leads you to the future and the belief that life can get better, so there becomes an optimism to feel peace again and the reality of future happiness. So what is there left to say? Only that hope can be found in the title of this book: **'THERE WILL ALWAYS BE A SUNRISE.'**

www.ingramcontent.com/pod-product-compliance
Lightning Source LLC
Chambersburg PA
CBHW031209270326
41931CB00006B/481